THE ENCYCLOPEDIA OF PSYCHOACTIVE DRUGS

SERIES 1

The Addictive Personality
Alcohol and Alcoholism
Alcohol Customs and Rituals
Alcohol Teenage Drinking
Amphetamines Danger in the Fast Lane
Barbiturates Sleeping Potion or Intoxicant?
Caffeine The Most Popular Stimulant
Cocaine A New Epidemic
Escape from Anxiety and Stress
Flowering Plants Magic in Bloom
Getting Help Treatments for Drug Abuse
Heroin The Street Narcotic
Inhalants The Toxic Fumes
LSD Visions or Nightmares?
Marijuana Its Effects on Mind & Body
Methadone Treatment for Addiction
Mushrooms Psychedelic Fungi
Nicotine An Old-Fashioned Addiction
Over-The-Counter Drugs Harmless or Hazardous?
PCP The Dangerous Angel
Prescription Narcotics The Addictive Painkillers
Quaaludes The Quest for Oblivion
Teenage Depression and Drugs
Treating Mental Illness
Valium and Other Tranquilizers

SERIES 2

Bad Trips
Brain Function
Case Histories
Celebrity Drug Use
Designer Drugs
The Downside of Drugs
Drinking, Driving, and Drugs
Drugs and Civilization
Drugs and Crime
Drugs and Diet
Drugs and Disease
Drugs and Emotion
Drugs and Pain
Drugs and Perception
Drugs and Pregnancy
Drugs and Sexual Behavior
Drugs and Sleep
Drugs and Sports
Drugs and the Arts
Drugs and the Brain
Drugs and the Family
Drugs and the Law
Drugs and Women
Drugs of the Future
Drugs Through the Ages
Drug Use Around the World
Legalization: A Debate
Mental Disturbances
Nutrition and the Brain
The Origins and Sources of Drugs
Substance Abuse: Prevention and Treatment
Who Uses Drugs?

DRUGS & THE BRAIN

THE ENCYCLOPEDIA OF PSYCHOACTIVE DRUGS

SERIES 2

DRUGS & THE BRAIN

EDWARD EDELSON

CHELSEA HOUSE PUBLISHERS
NEW YORK • PHILADELPHIA

EDITOR-IN-CHIEF: Nancy Toff
EXECUTIVE EDITOR: Remmel T. Nunn
MANAGING EDITOR: Karyn Gullen Browne
COPY CHIEF: Perry Scott King
ART DIRECTOR: Gianella Garrett
PICTURE EDITOR: Elizabeth Terhune

STAFF FOR DRUGS AND THE BRAIN:

SENIOR EDITOR: Jane Larkin Crain
ASSOCIATE EDITOR: Paula Edelson
ASSISTANT EDITOR: Michele A. Merens
DESIGNER: Victoria Tomaselli
COPY EDITORS: Sean Dolan, Gillian Bucky
CAPTIONS: Martin Baldessari
PICTURE RESEARCH: Matthew Miller
PRODUCTION COORDINATOR: Alma Rodriguez
PRODUCTION ASSISTANT: Karen Dreste

CREATIVE DIRECTOR: Harold Steinberg

COVER: Herbert Wagner/Phototake—NYC

Printed and bound in the United States of America

3 5 7 9 8 6 4

Library of Congress Cataloging-in-Publication Data
Edelson, Edward, 1932–
Drugs & the brain.
(The Encyclopedia of psychoactive drugs. Series 2)
Bibliography: p.
Includes index.
Summary: Examines the effects of both beneficial and potentially damaging psychoactive drugs on the human brain.
1. Psychotropic drugs—Juvenile literature. 2. Brain—Effect of drugs on—Juvenile literature. 3. Drug abuse—Physiological aspects—Juvenile literature. 4. Psychotropic drugs—Toxicology—Juvenile literature. [1. Psychotropic drugs. 2. Brain—Effect of drugs on. 3. Drugs] I. Title. II. Title: Drugs and the brain. III. Series.
RM315.E33 1987 615′.78 86-31764

ISBN 1-55546-209-X

0-7910-0796-0 (pbk.)

CONTENTS

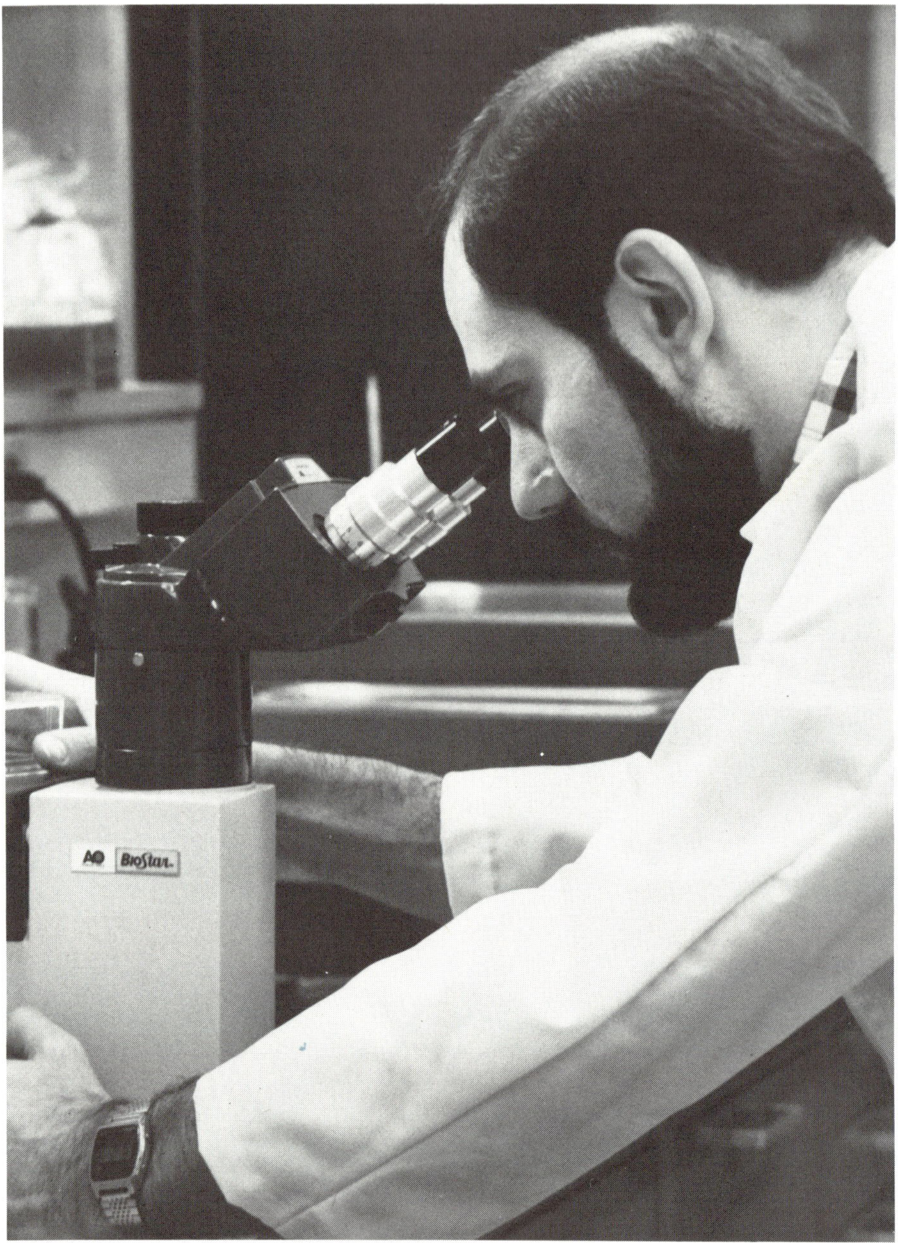

The contradictory and still largely unexplored effects that certain substances have on the human brain have inspired scientists around the world to establish laboratories such as this one. Scientists at these centers are conducting research to examine and document the ways different drugs affect brain functions.

FOREWORD

In the Mainstream of American Life

One of the legacies of the social upheaval of the 1960s is that psychoactive drugs have become part of the mainstream of American life. Schools, homes, and communities cannot be "drug proofed." There is a demand for drugs — and the supply is plentiful. Social norms have changed and drugs are not only available—they are everywhere.

But where efforts to curtail the supply of drugs and outlaw their use have had tragically limited effects on demand, it may be that education has begun to stem the rising tide of drug abuse among young people and adults alike.

Over the past 25 years, as drugs have become an increasingly routine facet of contemporary life, a great many teenagers have adopted the notion that drug taking was somehow a right or a privilege or a necessity. They have done so, however, without understanding the consequences of drug use during the crucial years of adolescence.

The teenage years are few in the total life cycle, but critical in the maturation process. During these years adolescents face the difficult tasks of discovering their identity, clarifying their sexual roles, asserting their independence, learning to cope with authority, and searching for goals that will give their lives meaning.

Drugs rob adolescents of precious time, stamina, and health. They interrupt critical learning processes, sometimes forever. Teenagers who use drugs are likely to withdraw increasingly into themselves, to "cop out" at just the time when they most need to reach out and experience the world.

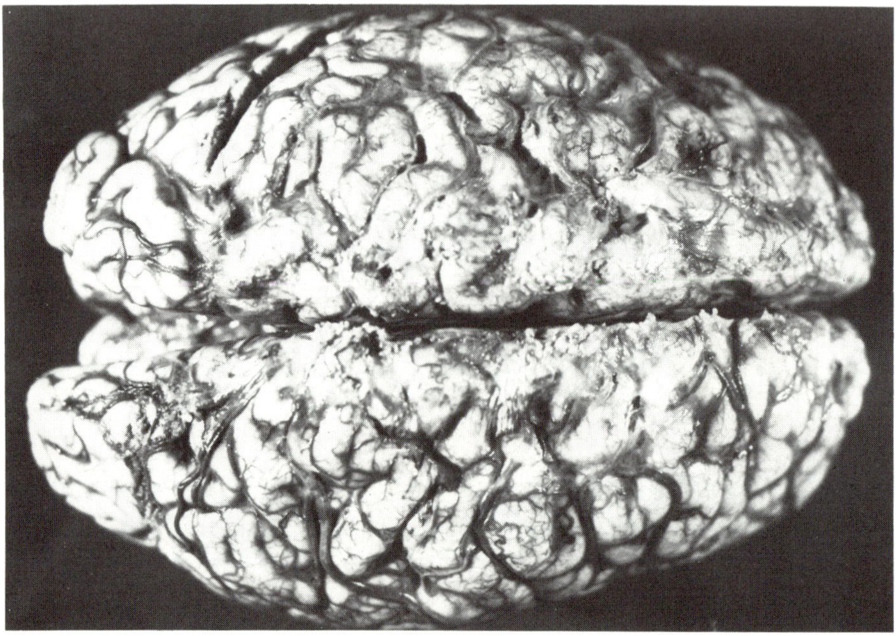

An overview of the human brain, the organ that regulates and coordinates all of the body's sensory and motor activities.

Fortunately, as a recent Gallup poll shows, young people are beginning to realize this, too. They themselves label drugs their most important problem. In the last few years, moreover, the climate of tolerance and ignorance surrounding drugs has been changing.

Adolescents as well as adults are becoming aware of mounting evidence that every race, ethnic group, and class is vulnerable to drug dependency.

Recent publicity about the cost and failure of drug rehabilitation efforts; dangerous drug use among pilots, air traffic controllers, star athletes, and Hollywood celebrities; and drug-related accidents, suicides, and violent crime have focused the public's attention on the need to wage an all-out war on drug abuse before it seriously undermines the fabric of society itself.

The anti-drug message is getting stronger and there is evidence that the message is beginning to get through to adults and teenagers alike.

The Enyclopedia of Psychoactive Drugs hopes to play a part in the national campaign now underway to educate young people about drugs. Series 1 provides clear and comprehensive discussions of common psychoactive substances, outlines their psychological and physiological effects on the mind and body, explains how they "hook" the user, and separates fact from myth in the complex issue of drug abuse.

Whereas Series 1 focuses on specific drugs, such as nicotine or cocaine, Series 2 confronts a broad range of both social and physiological phenomena. Each volume addresses the ramifications of drug use and abuse on some aspect of human experience: social, familial, cultural, historical, and physical. Separate volumes explore questions about the effects of drugs on brain chemistry and unborn children; the use and abuse of painkillers; the relationship between drugs and sexual behavior, sports, and the arts; drugs and disease; the role of drugs in history and the sophisticated drugs now being developed in the laboratory that will profoundly change the future.

Each book in the series is fully illustrated and is tailored to the needs and interests of young readers. The more adolescents know about drugs and their role in society, the less likely they are to misuse them.

Joann Rodgers
Senior Editorial Consultant

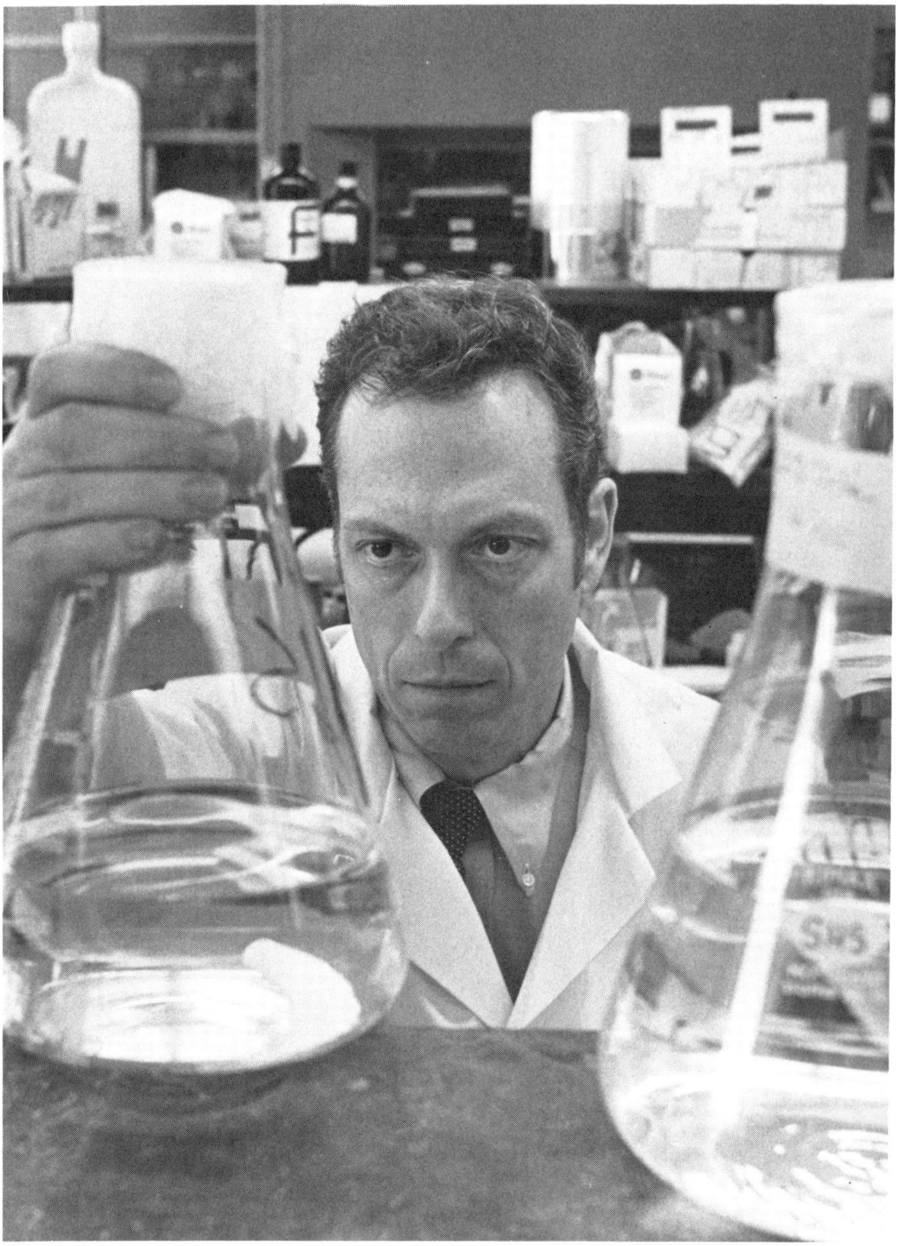

Dr. Solomon Snyder, a professor at Johns Hopkins University, was one of the first scientists to isolate and identify natural opiates in the human brain. The discovery of these opiates, which are called endorphins, could help unravel mysteries concerning how and why the human brain interacts with psychoactive drugs.

INTRODUCTION

The Gift of Wizardry
Use and Abuse

JACK H. MENDELSON, M.D.
NANCY K. MELLO, PH.D.
Alcohol and Drug Abuse Research Center
Harvard Medical School—McLean Hospital

Dorothy to the Wizard:

"I think you are a very bad man," said Dorothy.
"Oh no, my dear; I'm really a very good man; but I'm a very bad Wizard."

—from THE WIZARD OF OZ

Man is endowed with the gift of wizardry, a talent for discovery and invention. The discovery and invention of substances that change the way we feel and behave are among man's special accomplishments, and, like so many other products of our wizardry, these substances have the capacity to harm as well as to help. Psychoactive drugs can cause profound changes in the chemistry of the brain and other vital organs, and although their legitimate use can relieve pain and cure disease, their abuse leads in a tragic number of cases to destruction.

Consider alcohol — available to all and yet regarded with intense ambivalence from biblical times to the present day. The use of alcoholic beverages dates back to our earliest ancestors. Alcohol use and misuse became associated with the worship of gods and demons. One of the most powerful Greek gods was Dionysus, lord of fruitfulness and god of wine. The Romans adopted Dionysus but changed his name to Bacchus. Festivals and holidays associated with Bacchus celebrated the harvest and the origins of life. Time has blurred the images of the Bacchanalian festival, but the theme of drunkenness as a major part of celebration has survived the pagan gods and remains a familiar part of modern society. The term "Bacchanalian Festival" conveys a more appealing image than "drunken orgy" or "pot party," but whatever the label, drinking alcohol is a form of drug use that results in addiction for millions.

The fact that many millions of other people can use alcohol in moderation does not mitigate the toll this drug takes on society as a whole. According to reliable estimates, one out of every ten Americans develops a serious alcohol-related problem sometime in his or her lifetime. In addition, automobile accidents caused by drunken drivers claim the lives of tens of thousands every year. Many of the victims are gifted young people, just starting out in adult life. Hospital emergency rooms abound with patients seeking help for alcohol-related injuries.

Who is to blame? Can we blame the many manufacturers who produce such an amazing variety of alcoholic beverages? Should we blame the educators who fail to explain the perils of intoxication, or so exaggerate the dangers of drinking that no one could possibly believe them? Are friends to blame — those peers who urge others to "drink more and faster," or the macho types who stress the importance of being able to "hold your liquor"? Casting blame, however, is hardly constructive, and pointing the finger is a fruitless way to deal with the problem. Alcoholism and drug abuse have few culprits but many victims. Accountability begins with each of us, every time we choose to use or misuse an intoxicating substance.

It is ironic that some of man's earliest medicines, derived from natural plant products, are used today to poison and to intoxicate. Relief from pain and suffering is one of society's many continuing goals. Over 3,000 years ago, the Therapeutic Papyrus of Thebes, one of our earliest written records, gave instructions for the use of opium in the treatment of pain. Opium, in the form of its major derivative, morphine, and similar compounds, such as heroin, have also been used by many to induce changes in mood and feeling. Another example of man's misuse of a natural substance is the coca leaf, which for centuries was used by the Indians of Peru to reduce fatigue and hunger. Its modern derivative, cocaine, has important medical use as a local anesthetic. Unfortunately, its increasing abuse in the 1980s clearly has reached epidemic proportions.

The purpose of this series is to explore in depth the psychological and behavioral effects that psychoactive drugs have on the individual, and also, to investigate the ways in which drug use influences the legal, economic, cultural, and even moral aspects of societies. The information presented here (and in other books in this series) is based on many clinical and laboratory studies and other observations by people from diverse walks of life.

Over the centuries, novelists, poets, and dramatists have provided us with many insights into the sometimes seductive but ultimately problematic aspects of alcohol and drug use. Physicians, lawyers, biologists, psychologists, and social scientists have contributed to a better understanding of the causes and consequences of using these substances. The authors in this series have attempted to gather and condense all the latest information about drug use and abuse. They have also described the sometimes wide gaps in our knowledge and have suggested some new ways to answer many difficult questions.

One such question, for example, is how do alcohol and drug problems get started? And what is the best way to treat them when they do? Not too many years ago, alcoholics and drug abusers were regarded as evil, immoral, or both. It is now recognized that these persons suffer from very complicated diseases involving deep psychological and social problems. To understand how the disease begins and progresses, it is necessary to understand the nature of the substance, the behavior of addicts, and the characteristics of the society or culture in which they live.

Although many of the social environments we live in are very similar, some of the most subtle differences can strongly influence our thinking and behavior. Where we live, go to school and work, whom we discuss things with — all influence our opinions about drug use and misuse. Yet we also share certain commonly accepted beliefs that outweigh any differences in our attitudes. The authors in this series have tried to identify and discuss the central, most crucial issues concerning drug use and misuse.

Despite the increasing sophistication of the chemical substances we create in the laboratory, we have a long way to go in our efforts to make these powerful drugs work for us rather than against us.

The volumes in this series address a wide range of timely questions. What influence has drug use had on the arts? Why do so many of today's celebrities and star athletes use drugs, and what is being done to solve this problem? What is the relationship between drugs and crime? What is the physiological basis for the power drugs can hold over us? These are but a few of the issues explored in this far-ranging series.

Educating people about the dangers of drugs can go a long way towards minimizing the desperate consequences of substance abuse for individuals and society as a whole. Luckily, human beings have the resources to solve even the most serious problems that beset them, once they make the commitment to do so. As one keen and sensitive observer, Dr. Lewis Thomas, has said,

> There is nothing at all absurd about the human condition. We matter. It seems to me a good guess, hazarded by a good many people who have thought about it, that we may be engaged in the formation of something like a mind for the life of this planet. If this is so, we are still at the most primitive stage, still fumbling with language and thinking, but infinitely capacitated for the future. Looked at this way, it is remarkable that we've come as far as we have in so short a period, really no time at all as geologists measure time. We are the newest, youngest, and the brightest thing around.

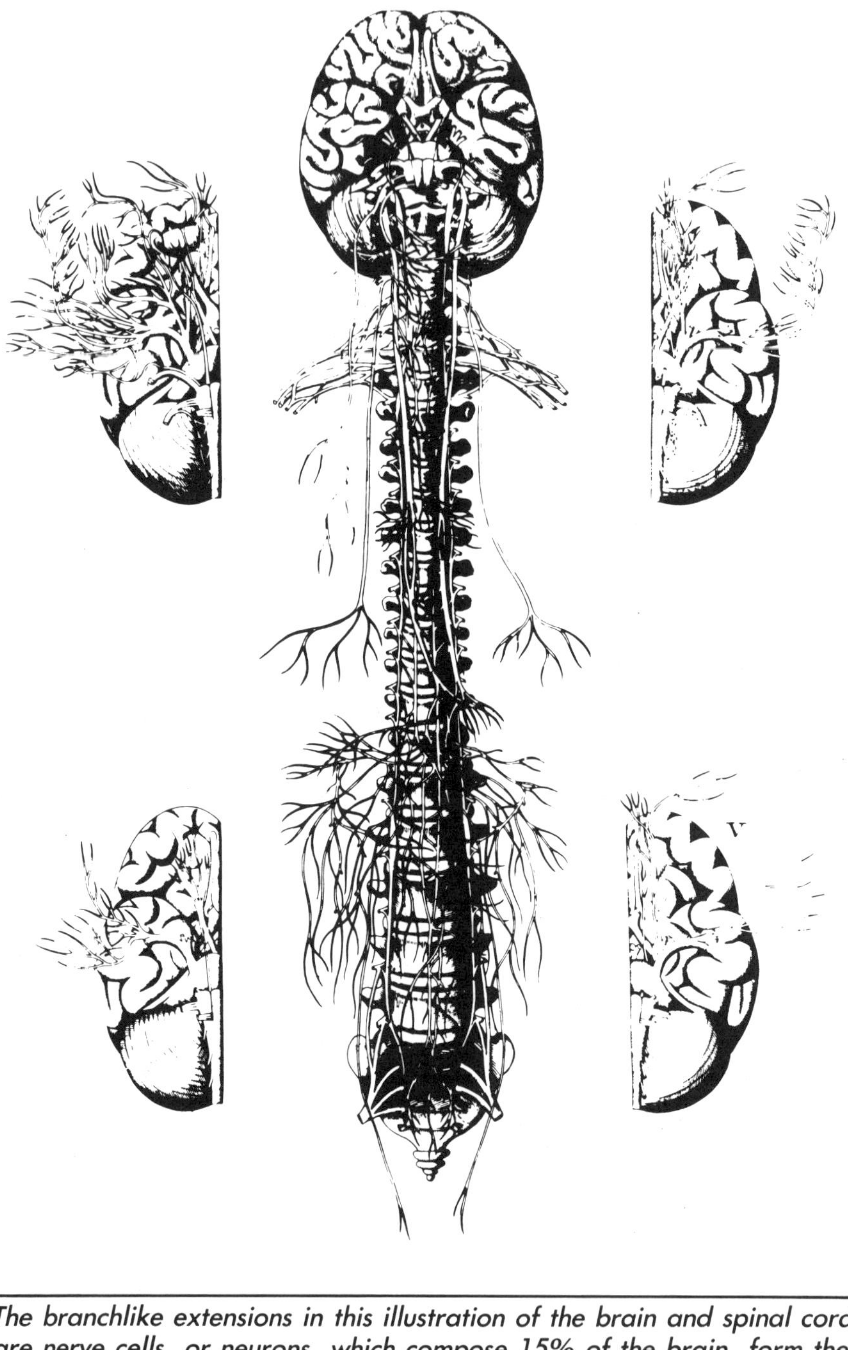

The branchlike extensions in this illustration of the brain and spinal cord are nerve cells, or neurons, which compose 15% of the brain, form the spinal cord, and fan out to every part of the body.

CHAPTER 1

HOW THE BRAIN WORKS

By definition, psychoactive drugs affect the way the brain works — for better or for worse. They can make us more alert, sedate us, produce strange mental pictures, ease our sensation of pain, disorient our normal ways of thinking, or restore some disoriented ways of thinking to normal. Some of them are among the most beneficial drugs known to medicine. Some are among the most damaging in our society.

The use of psychoactive drugs is nearly as old as the human race. Alcohol, for example, appears to have been with us in the earliest days of civilization. Opiates (compounds including morphine, codeine, and their derivatives, such as heroin) have been known for thousands of years. Other drugs are very recent productions, synthesized in laboratories in the past decades or even in the past few years. One of the extraordinary scientific feats of this century is the discovery of whole new classes of drugs that affect the operation of the human mind. An even greater accomplishment has been to find out how psychoactive drugs produce their remarkable effects.

Clues Hidden Within the Brain

The two achievements go hand in hand. By studying psychoactive drugs, scientists learn more about the way the brain works. They can use that knowledge to produce psychoactive drugs that are more effective. The beneficial results of this work are all around us: new drugs have been used to relieve anxiety, ease depression, and allow many patients with schizophrenia to lead normal lives. The adverse effects of this knowledge are also omnipresent: there has been a huge increase in the number of bootleg drugs made in home laboratories for illegal street use.

Many psychoactive drugs were discovered accidentally, but modern neuroscientists have been quick to capitalize on those accidents. One outstanding example is drug treatment of depression. Researchers stumbled across the first antidepressant drugs through a series of lucky coincidences, which we will discuss later in this volume. By analyzing the way those drugs worked, scientists have been able to create whole families of antidepressants.

The key to such advances is knowledge about the brain — about the cells that make up this remarkable 3-lb biological computer and about the organization that makes the brain superior to any digital computer that human ingenuity has yet been able to manufacture.

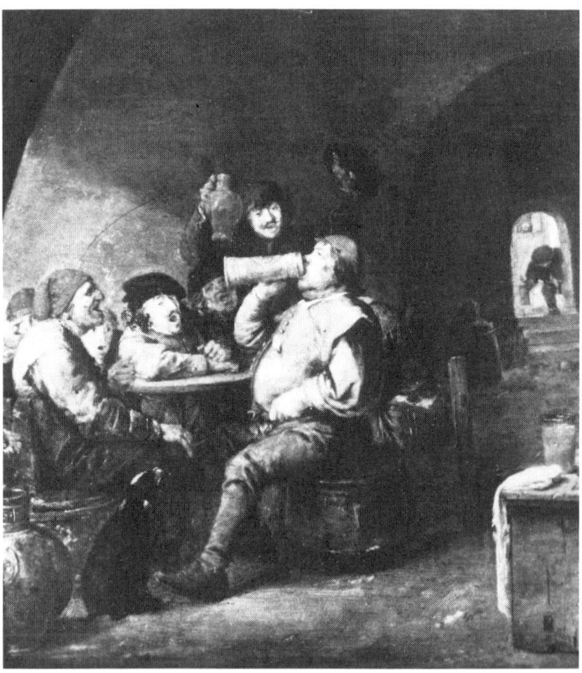

Peasants drink wine in this 17th-century painting by the Dutch artist Adrian Brouwer. Although the use of alcohol is nearly as old as mankind, the effects of this drug on the human mind and body are still being explored.

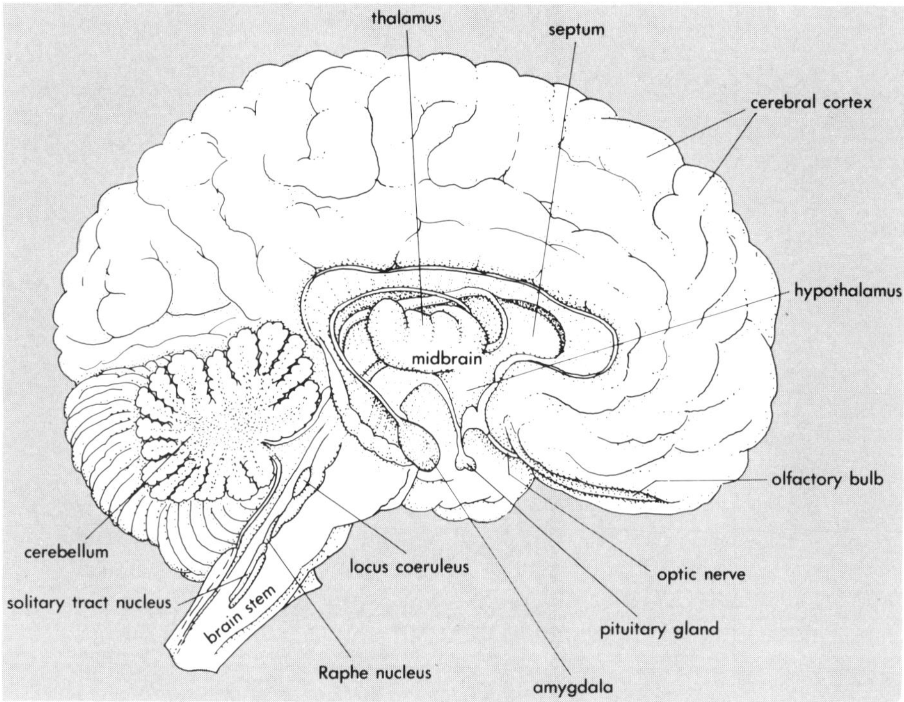

A cross section of the brain shows its three main regions: the cerebral cortex, the midbrain, and the brain stem. Other major regions of the brain are also indicated.

For centuries anatomists have studied the visible features of the brain. They have identified and named structures large and small in the brain's two hemispheres. More recently, neuroscientists have begun to understand the fine workings of the brain. One of the most important things they have learned is how individual brain cells transmit signals to one another — not by using electrical impulses, as was once thought, but by sending bursts of chemicals across the space between nerve cells.

Neuroscientists can describe the activity of many drugs on the molecular level in terms of the way a given drug affects the transmission of chemical signals from one nerve cell to another. But the molecular picture is only the beginning of the story. To understand why one drug makes us sleepy and eases pain while another makes us feel abnormally alert, we have to look at the major structures of the brain and the nerve cells of which they are composed.

Neurons and Glia

The brain has two major kinds of cells: *neurons* and *glia*. About 85% of brain cells are glia. They seem to play a supporting role in brain function, guiding its development and helping to remove waste products. It is the other 15% of brain cells, the neurons, that make the brain what it is — the organ that not only controls the body's essential activities and emotions, but also gives humans their unique power to think.

Neurons are nerve cells. The neurons of the brain are no different in basic structure from those that run down to form the spinal cord and fan out to every part of the body. Like other cells, a neuron has a main cell body. This body is composed of a nucleus, which contains the genetic material that allows a cell to reproduce, and a surrounding portion called the cytoplasm, which contains the structures that provide energy for the cell. Unlike other cells, a neuron has thin extensions that can be extremely long — up to 4 feet long in a human, 15 feet in a giraffe. These extensions are called *axons*. They are essential links that allow neurons to communicate with one another.

At the end of an axon are thousands of tiny branches, each of which can make contact with another neuron. Sometimes an axon of one neuron reaches out to the cell body of another neuron. More often, an axon makes contact with a shorter extension of a neighboring neuron, called a *dendrite*. A single neuron can have many axons and more than 10,000 dendrites, each capable of receiving signals from many other neurons.

The Ultimate in Data Processing

The human brain controls about 10 billion neurons — a number that sounds impressive but is really small considering the phenomenal amount of data processing that the brain does routinely. The largest, fastest digital computer, working at top speed, cannot process information as efficiently and intelligently as the human brain — as, for example, when we return a tough tennis shot, rapidly assessing many variables and exercising the higher powers of reason that are unique to human beings. It is not so much the number of neurons in the brain as their interconnections that are responsible for that data-processing ability. The multiplicity and complexity of the connections between neurons in the brain give us the capabilities that make us human beings.

The picture of an individual neuron — say, one that transmits a pain signal — is rather simple. When you prick yourself with a pin and stimulate a pain nerve, an electrical signal runs down its axon. A nerve cell has an outer wall, a membrane, which is full of a fluid that contains salts, including sodium, potassium, and chloride ions. All of them are electrically charged particles. The membrane is surrounded by body fluid that also contains charged particles.

At rest, the interior of the neuron has a greater electrical charge than the fluid surrounding it. When the neuron is stimulated by the pinprick, its membrane allows a large quantity of positively charged sodium ions to enter the cell at the point of stimulation. This inrush of sodium ions at the point of stimulation changes the properties of the neighboring part of the membrane, allowing sodium ions to enter there as well. The result is a wave of electrochemical activity that moves rapidly down the neuron, much as an electrical current runs down a wire.

When you prick your finger, the nerve that is stimulated does not carry the pain signal directly to the brain. Instead, it passes the message along to another neuron, and so on, until the signal reaches the brain. For decades neuroscientists were puzzled about how the nerve cells pass signals from one nerve cell to another. Only in the last 40 years or so have they learned that nerve cells communicate by transmitting chemical signals.

Neurotransmitters and Drug Actions

When the impulse caused by the inrush of sodium ions reaches the end of a neuron, it releases a chemical that passes across the narrow gap to a neighboring neuron. The gap is called a *synapse* and the chemical is called a *neurotransmitter*. Sometimes a neurotransmitter causes the neighboring nerve to fire. Sometimes it prevents the neighboring nerve from firing. A single neuron can easily be in contact with hundreds of other neurons, some of which stimulate it to act and others that inhibit its action.

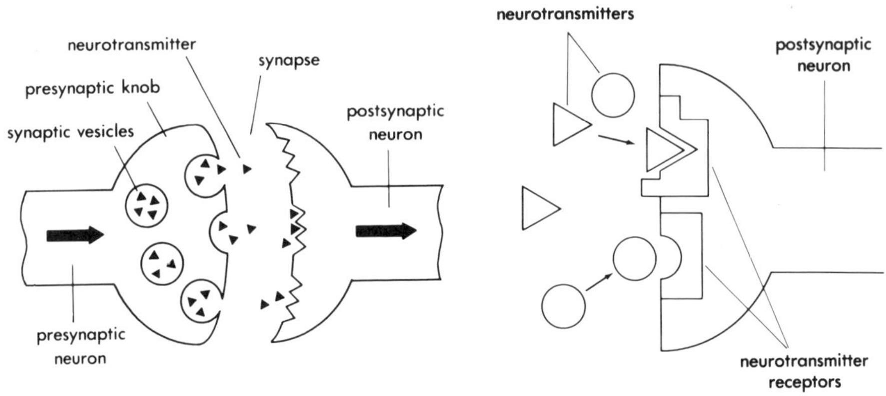

The drawing on the left shows how one neuron signals another across the synapse between them by emitting neurotransmitters. The illustration on the right shows how each kind of neurotransmitter fits only one kind of receptor on the target neuron.

A neurotransmitter from one nerve cell acts on the neighboring cell by attaching itself to a specific molecule in that cell's membrane. That molecule is called a *receptor*. Each receptor recognizes only one neurotransmitter. We can think of a receptor as a lock that is precision made to be opened only by one key.

As soon as a neurotransmitter acts on a receptor, the neurotransmitter is removed from action in one of several ways: some neurotransmitters are destroyed by enzymes, but most are absorbed back into the neuron that released them. A few are absorbed by glia.

There are a number of ways drugs can interact with the neurotransmitter system to alter brain activity. Some drugs prevent the formation of neurotransmitters. Others cause neurotransmitters to leak out of a nerve-cell ending. Still other drugs increase the activity of neurotransmitters, either by inhibiting the enzymes that destroy them or by preventing them from being reabsorbed by the nerve that emits them.

The most common way a drug affects neurotransmitter

activity is by influencing receptors. Some psychoactive drugs produce the same effects as a neurotransmitter because they can fit into the receptor, triggering the cell into activity. Others block neurotransmitter activity because they fit into receptors and deactivate the neurotransmitter.

Brain Sites of Drug Actions

Just as important as how a drug or a neurotransmitter operates is where in the brain it has its effect. Specific neurotransmitters tend to be associated with specific brain centers, or with circuits of neurons that direct the activity of different brain centers. The discovery of neurotransmitters goes hand in hand with studies examining where in the brain they act.

The human brain can be divided into three main parts: the *forebrain*, or *cerebral cortex*, which governs higher functions such as thought and language; the *midbrain*, which controls such necessary functions as breathing; and the *brain stem*, which regulates the most primitive functions.

The brain can be subdivided into many more regions: the *extrapyramidal areas*, below the cerebral cortex, which control movement; the *limbic system*, which sorts out meaningful signals from the perceptions that flood the brain; and still others. Neuroscientists have learned a lot about the interactions among these brain centers, but they still have much more to learn. One major way they learn is by studying neurotransmitter activity.

Acetylcholine

The first neurotransmitter discovered was *acetylcholine*, which was isolated in the 1920s from nerves that regulate heart function. The story began in 1921 with experiments by a German scientist, Otto Loewi, on the *vagus nerve,* which runs from the brain stem to various parts of the body, including the heart. One of its effects is to slow the heartbeat. Loewi placed a frog's heart in a fluid solution and electrically stimulated it to make it beat. He then stimulated the vagus nerve, and the heart stopped beating. When he exposed another frog's heart to the same fluid, it also stopped beating, an indication that a chemical released by the vagus nerve was in the fluid and acted on the heart.

It took five years for Loewi to isolate acetylcholine and to show that it is the chemical that the vagus nerve releases. It took another decade for researchers to work out how the body makes acetylcholine: a molecule of *choline*, which is found in many foods, is linked to a molecule of *acetylcoenzyme A*, a form of acetic acid, which is found in vinegar.

Other researchers found that acetylcholine is stored in tiny vessels called *synaptic vesicles*, which are located at the end of the axon. After acetylcholine is released and acts on the neighboring nerve, an enzyme called *acetylcholinesterase* destroys the neurotransmitter by breaking it into choline and acetic acid. The inactivation of acetylcholine by an enzyme makes it unusual, because most other neurotransmitters are inactivated by being absorbed back into the emitting neuron. In other respects, however, acetylcholine is a model for all other neurotransmitters.

Research on acetylcholine has had many practical effects. Acetylcholine is not only the neurotransmitter for more than 10% of the nerves in the human body but is also found in many animals, including insects. Some of the most widely used insecticides kill pests by interfering with the activity of acetylcholinesterase, the enzyme that destroys acetylcholine. Because the insecticides contain this enzyme, they can also poison humans.

In addition to affecting the heart, acetylcholine acts upon structures in the cerebral cortex, where it appears to play a major role in the nerve centers for thought and higher mental functions. It is known that marijuana smoking causes changes in brain chemistry that inhibit acetylcholine, which transfers information from one nerve cell to another. This may explain marijuana's effects on memory and other mental processes. Destruction of nerves that use acetylcholine has also been linked with the development of *Alzheimer's disease*, a progressive disease (one that grows increasingly severe) that involves an irreversible loss of memory and deterioration of other intellectual functions. Researchers are now attempting to develop drugs that will ease the symptoms of Alzheimer's disease by substituting for the missing acetylcholine.

The work that has been done on finding a cure for Alzheimer's disease illustrates the sweeping nature of neurotransmitter research. Scientists were led to the link between Alzheimer's disease and acetylcholine by earlier studies on drugs called *belladonna alkaloids*, which are extracted from the belladonna plant. These drugs have been used as poisons in the past. Large doses can cause loss of memory and other mental functions and can be fatal.

In the 1930s researchers showed that a drug called *atropine*, the active ingredient of the belladonna plant, produces its effect by blocking an acetylcholine receptor. In the 1980s the realization that belladonna poisoning produces effects similar to those of Alzheimer's disease led to more research concerning acetylcholine.

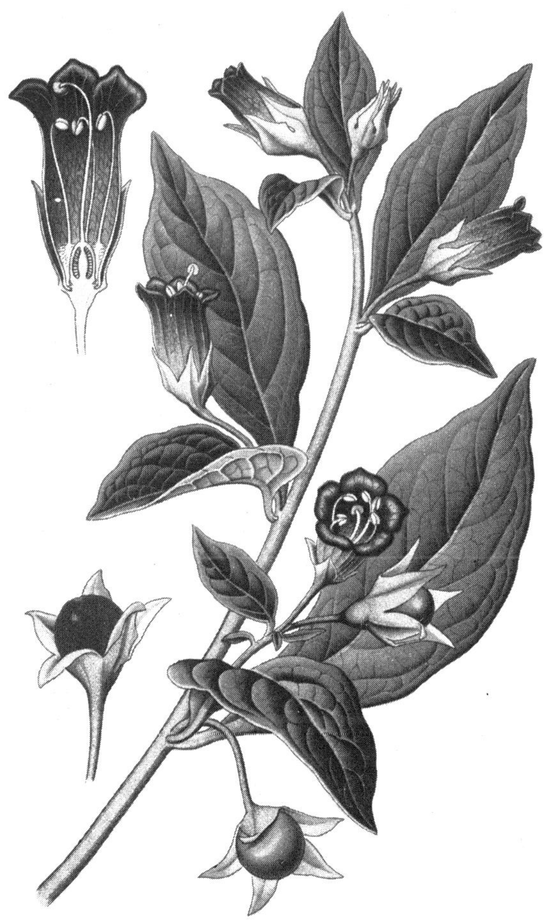

When an active ingredient in the belladonna plant blocks the acetylcholine receptors in the human body, loss of memory and other mental dysfunctions occur. These effects are similar to those of Alzheimer's disease, a progressive illness that until recently was often mistaken for senility. Research is now being undertaken on possible links between acetylcholine depletion and Alzheimer's disease.

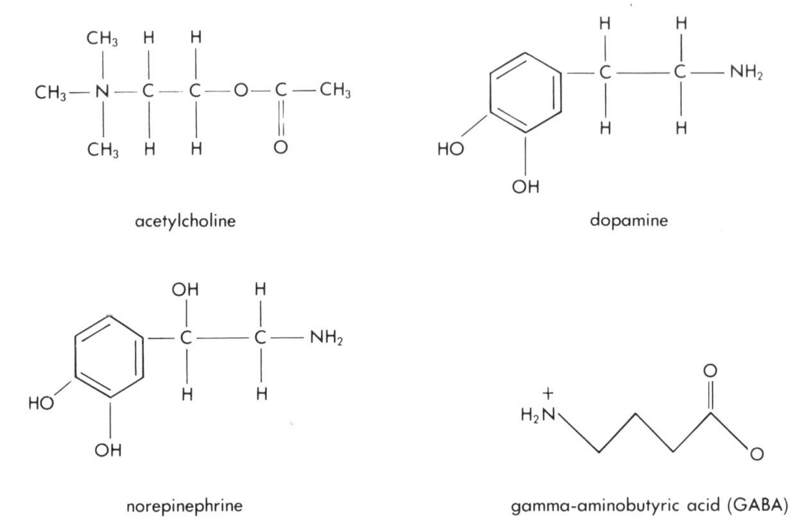

The chemical structures of four neurotransmitters. Some psychoactive drugs produce their effects by increasing the activity of neurotransmitters, others by preventing their normal formation in neurons.

Norepinephrine

The second neurotransmitter to be discovered was *norepinephrine*, which was isolated in the 1930s. It is found in the *autonomic nervous system* (the part of the nervous system concerned with control of involuntary bodily functions), which is responsible for the "fight or flight" response to emergencies — faster heartbeat, elevation of blood pressure and so on. Chemically, norepinephrine is a *catecholamine*, a class of compounds that affects the nervous and cardiovascular systems, metabolic rate, and body temperature.

Dopamine

Dopamine, another catecholamine, was identified as a neurotransmitter in the late 1950s. One of the places that it acts in is the *corpus striatum*, a part of the brain that regulates motor behavior. The most significant advance ever made in the treatment of Parkinson's disease — a degenerative condition whose symptoms include muscle rigidity and tremors and difficulty in moving — was made possible by the discovery that neurons that use dopamine are destroyed in patients who have this disease. The standard treatment for Parkinson's disease involves the administration of a drug called L-dopa, which is transformed into dopamine in the brain. An illustration of the complexity of brain function is the fact that excess dopamine activity in another part of the brain, the limbic system, has been found in patients with schizophrenia. Because of this connection, drugs that relieve the symptoms of schizophrenia can also cause Parkinsonlike symptoms.

Newly Discovered Neurotransmitters

The number of known neurotransmitters has multiplied in the past decade. More than 50 have been discovered, and new ones are constantly identified. Some of them are amino acids, compounds that are linked together to form proteins, which are essential for the growth and repair of the body's tissues. One amino acid, glycine, is a neurotransmitter in the spinal cord and brain stem. Another, glutamic acid, is found in neurons that connect the cerebral cortex and the corpus striatum. *Gamma-aminobutyric acid* (GABA) is an amino acid neurotransmitter that acts on anywhere from 25% to 40% of all brain synapses. It is an *inhibitory neurotransmitter*, meaning that it acts to reduce the rate of firing of neurons.

A large number of the newly discovered neurotransmitters are proteins, some small, some large. *Substance P*, a protein with 11 amino acids, is a neurotransmitter found in pain neurons and in several brain centers. *Endorphins*, newly discovered molecules that are the brain's natural opiates, are also proteins.

The discovery of natural opiates in the brain was one of the most significant events in modern neuroscience. It answered centuries-old questions about drugs that have helped and harmed us profoundly: the opiates. These drugs are discussed in Chapter 2.

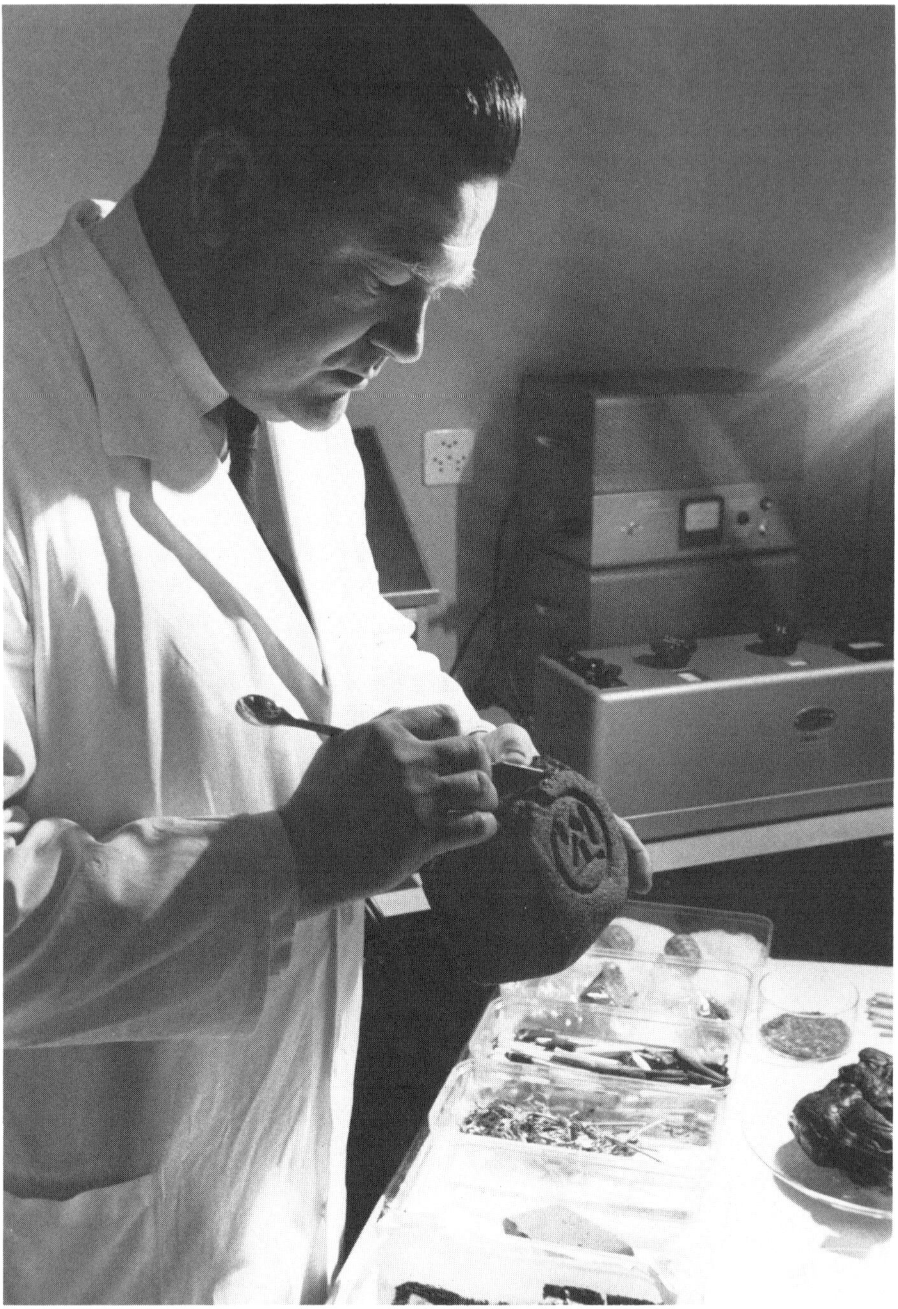

A scientist examines opium samples. Opiates, which have been used for medicinal purposes since ancient times, are also dangerously addictive and potentially fatal drugs of abuse.

CHAPTER 2

OPIATES AND THE BRAIN

The human race has known opiates (substances derived from opium) almost since the beginning of recorded history. Opium, an extract of the poppy plant, appears to have been used to relieve pain in the ancient Middle Eastern region of Sumeria as early as 4000 B.C.E. (B.C.E. stands for "before the common era" and is equivalent to B.C.; C.E., "common era," is used in place of A.D.) Galen, the great 2nd-century C.E. Greek physician, used opium as a treatment for asthma and heart disease. Even in the modern era, after centuries of research, nothing as effective as opiates for relieving extreme pain has been discovered.

Yet opiates are a double-edged sword. In addition to their valuable medical uses, they are the classic drugs of abuse. They offer a deceptive, temporary sense of well-being and euphoria that requires larger and larger doses to maintain. In addition, an opiate user who stops taking these drugs can suffer terrible withdrawal symptoms.

Painkiller or Intoxicant?

The romantic view of opiates was given in the 19th century by Thomas De Quincey, author of *Confessions of an English Opium-Eater*, who claimed that opium was "the secret of happiness" and described how "potable [drinkable] ecstasies might be corked up in a pint bottle and peace of mind could be sent down by the mail." But at about the same time, a British physician, John Jones, was describing what could happen to those who sought De Quincey's ecstasies. Those who suddenly stopped using opium, wrote Jones, experienced "great and even intolerable distresses, anxieties and depression of spirit which commonly end in a miserable death, attended with strange agonies, unless men return to the use of opium."

The medical and scientific history of the opiates consists of a long struggle to separate the marvelous pain-relieving qualities of these drugs from their ability to cause the kind of addiction described by Jones. Time after time, researchers have claimed the discovery of opiates that were effective against pain yet did not cause addiction. Time after time, the initial enthusiasm has ended in disappointment. The most ironic note in this history is that heroin, the most widely abused opiate today, was originally introduced as a nonaddictive substitute for morphine, another opiate.

Morphine, the main component of opium, was first isolated from the poppy plant in 1805 by a German chemist, Friedrich Serteurner, who named it after Morpheus, the Greek

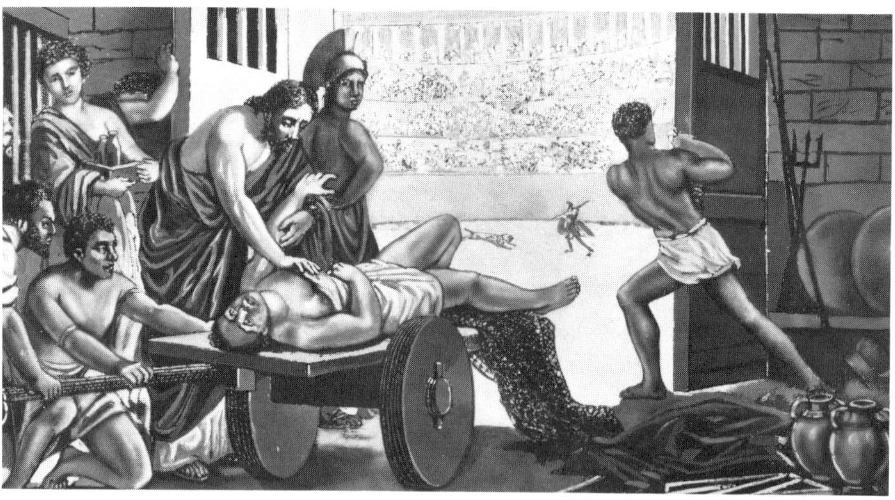

A drawing depicts Galen, the famous 2nd-century C.E. Greek physician, tending a wounded gladiator. Galen prescribed opium as a medication for such ailments as asthma and heart disease.

god of dreams. Chemists have since been able to make other opiates in the laboratory by modifying the morphine molecule. Heroin, for example, is made by adding two acetyl groups to the morphine molecule. Those added chemical groups enable heroin to dissolve quickly in the brain tissue, causing the "rush" that addicts crave.

Although scientists have worked with morphine and its relatives for well over a century, it is only in the past two decades that they have been able to determine why and how these drugs act as they do on the molecular level. Research concerning how opiates affect the brain is in many ways a model for the study of other psychoactive drugs.

Opiate Receptors and Antagonists

The research began with the basic assumption that opiates act on specific receptors in nerve cells. This assumption was based partly on previous knowledge gained about the functions of the *opiate antagonists*, which are drugs developed by chemists that counter the effects of opiates. Chemically, opiates and opiate antagonists have similar structures. Yet opiate antagonists have none of the effects of opiates — no euphoria, no pain relief. Instead, opiate antagonists are used to reverse swiftly the effects of opiates. Medically, opiate antagonists can be useful. An overdose of heroin or another opiate can cause death by shutting down the body's breathing apparatus. An injection of one well-known opiate antagonist, naloxone, can bring someone who has suffered a heroin overdose out of a deep coma to near-normal alertness in less than a minute. That response can be thought of as the result of a competition for the opiate receptors, a competition that the opiate antagonists win. In a startlingly brief time, the antagonist molecules are able to displace the opiate molecules from all receptors, canceling their effects.

In principle, the search for opiate receptors in the brain is simple. The researcher takes a sample of brain tissue, processes it to isolate the nerve-cell membranes that contain the receptors, and then adds an opiate that has been tagged (chemically attached) with a radioactive element. Using equipment that detects small amounts of radioactivity, the researcher then seeks the sites to which the radioactive opiates have become bound. Those sites should be the opiate receptors.

In practice, the search proved extremely difficult, partly because of the complex nature of brain-cell membranes, partly because opiates can also bind to molecules that are not receptors, and partly because opiate receptors are rather scarce in the brain. But in 1973, researchers at New York University, at Johns Hopkins University in Baltimore, and at Uppsala University in Sweden were able to isolate opiate receptors by employing a variety of careful techniques, including the use of naloxone molecules tagged with an extremely high level of radioactivity. Although few of the molecules bound to receptors, the molecules that did helped researchers identify and locate opiate receptors.

Discovery of these receptors opened the way for answers to a number of fascinating questions, the most interesting of which was: How do opiates produce their distinctive effects? The answer had two parts: one concerned the locations in the brain where opiates act; the other concerned the action of these opiates in the brain.

The Brain's Own Opiates

Research on the second issue was defined by a second question: Why should morphine, a chemical produced by a plant, act on human brain cells? Apparently, morphine and the other opiates resembled molecules produced in the brain. Two teams of researchers, one in Aberdeen, Scotland, and one in Baltimore, followed different paths to identify the brain's own opiates.

In Aberdeen, John Hughes and Hans Kosterlitz worked with tissue from the intestines, because opiates are known to inhibit the contraction of intestinal muscles (they are often used to treat diarrhea for this reason). In Baltimore, Solomon Snyder, Gavril Pasternak, and Rabi Simantov worked with brain tissue. Hughes and Kosterlitz were the first to identify natural brain opiates — two small protein molecules that they called *enkephalins*, from the Greek for "in the head." Not long afterward, the Baltimore researchers found the same brain opiates. Many scientists refer to these molecules as endorphins, and the two terms are now used interchangeably. Over the years, investigators have identified a large number of endorphins of varying potencies and different sites of action, as well as a number of different opiate receptors.

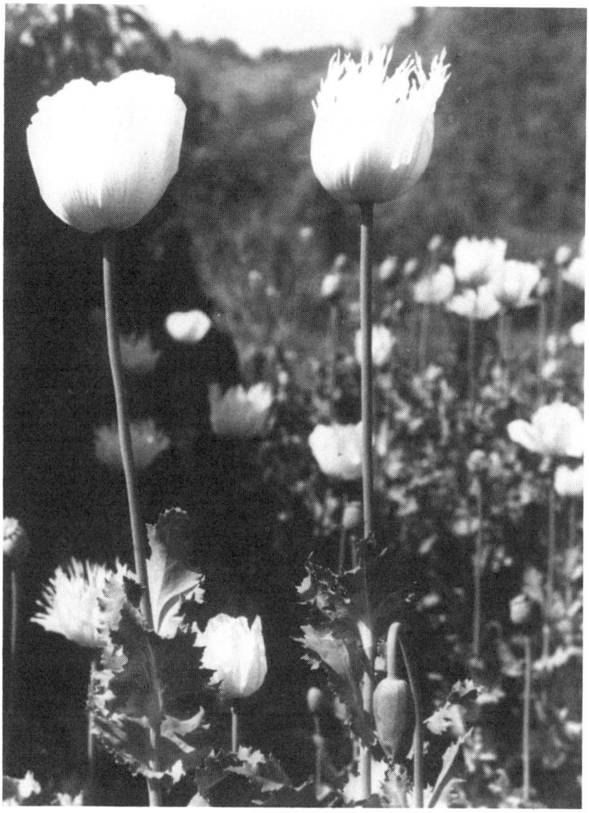

An opium poppy field in Thailand. Derivatives of opium, such as morphine and heroin, are produced from the dried juice of these plants.

Soon after the initial discovery was made, a number of neuroscientists were able to show that endorphins are neurotransmitters. They are released by neurons and produce their effects by either triggering or inhibiting the activity of other neurons. Having demonstrated this fact, the researchers could then turn their attention to explaining the reasons for the peculiar combination of opiate activities. They did this by looking at the areas in the brain and spinal cord where opiate receptors are found.

Employing a method developed at Johns Hopkins, Snyder, Michael Kuhar, and Candace Pert used radioactively tagged opiates to pinpoint the parts of the central nervous system where opiates are bound to receptors. As might have been expected, the areas where opiate receptors were most common were those involved with the perception of pain.

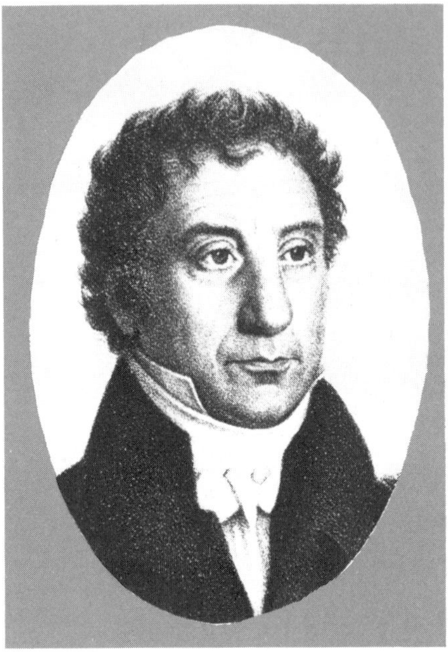

The German chemist Friedrich Serteurner identified morphine as the active ingredient in opium by isolating this drug from the poppy plant in the early 19th century.

Opiates relieve pain in an odd way — not by eliminating the pain but by making someone indifferent to it. Patients who are given morphine often remark that they can still feel the pain but that they are no longer bothered by it. The reason for this reaction is that the morphine acts not on the nerves that transmit pain sensations to the brain but on centers in the brain and spinal cord that integrate all incoming information about pain.

Snyder, Kuhar, and Pert found a high concentration of opiate receptors in the *substantia gelatinosa*, which is where pain nerves make their first contact with the spinal cord. They also found many opiate receptors in a brain structure called the *thalamus*, which handles input about deep, lasting, burning pain, the kind that opiates work best against. In the midbrain, opiate receptors were found in an area called the *periaqueductal gray zone*, where pain signals are processed.

The location of opiate receptors in the brain explained the causes of some of the non-pain-associated effects of these drugs. For example, heroin addicts can be easily identified by the constricted, "pinpoint" pupils of their eyes. A dense concentration of opiate receptors was found in the *pretectal nuclei*, located in the brain structure that controls pupil size. Opiates can kill by depressing (inhibiting) respiration until breathing is stopped because there are many opiate receptors in one of the major brain areas that control breathing — the *nucleus solitary tract*.

Perhaps the most intriguing concentration of opiate receptors was found in the part of the brain called the limbic system, the ring-shaped group of structures that runs around the brain stem just below the cerebral cortex. One logical explanation for the euphoric effect of opiates is that they act on the limbic system, the area of the brain that controls emotional behavior. This theory is not proven yet; neuroscientists still have incomplete information about the relationship between specific parts of the limbic system and emotional states such as euphoria. Such information is difficult to obtain from animal studies because emotions are so particularly human, but research on the subject continues.

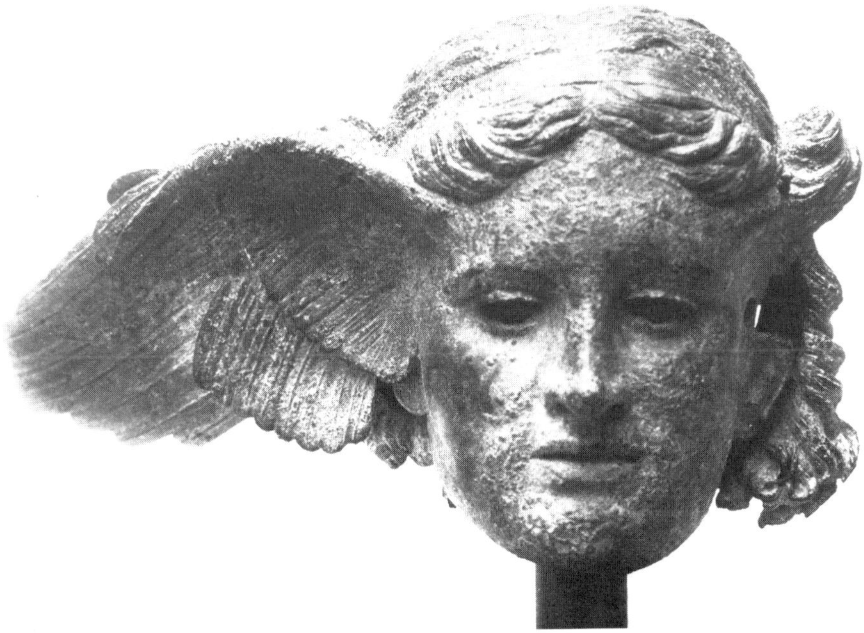

This 4th-century B.C.E. marble head with its heavy-lidded eyes is a representation of Morpheus, the Greek god of dreams, after whom morphine, the sedating narcotic, was named.

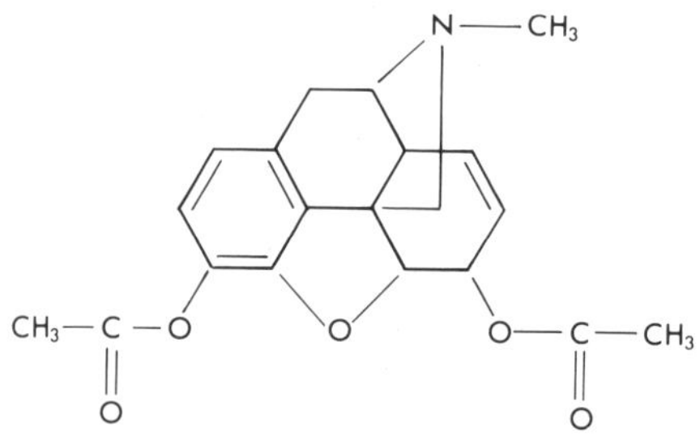

heroin

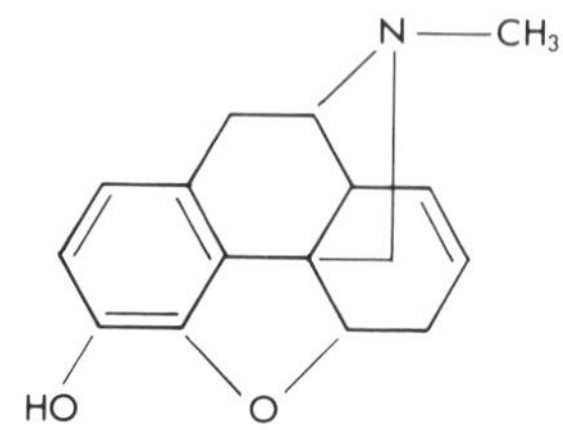

morphine

Heroin differs from morphine in that it has two additional acetyl groups in its chemical structure. Ironically, heroin was created as a result of continuing attempts to create a substance that had morphine's painkilling power but not its addictive properties.

Opiate Addiction

Research on opiate receptors and the brain's natural opiates has led to a convincing explanation of the causes behind other human responses to opiates, especially those involved in addiction. Drug addiction is a complex phenomenon that includes psychological factors, but it does have two physical components. One is *tolerance*, the need to take increasing doses of a drug to achieve the same effects experienced previously. The second is *physical dependence* — the body's craving for a drug — which causes withdrawal symptoms when the drug is stopped. The withdrawal symptoms of opiate addiction include agitation, sleeplessness, depression, unusual sensitivity to pain, stomach cramps, and diarrhea.

Several studies have indicated that both tolerance and physical dependence can occur in normal individuals not addicted to opiates if they engage in activities that increase the production of the body's natural opiates. Endorphins appear to be released as part of the body's normal response to physical exertion. Some researchers have suggested that increased production of endorphins causes "runner's high," the feeling of euphoria reported by people who run or jog regularly. It has also been suggested that runners who suddenly stop their regular exercise may experience the same withdrawal symptoms as heroin addicts, but in a milder form.

An explanation of the physical side of opiate addiction starts with the belief that the nerve cells in the brain are normally exposed to a steady concentration of endorphins. Morphine or other outside opiates bind to opiate receptors in the brain, causing the body to cut back its production of endorphins. Tolerance occurs over time because the normal production of endorphins stops, and the body then requires more and more of the outside opiates to meet its needs.

According to this model, when the drug is no longer taken, withdrawal symptoms occur because the body needs some time to resume production of its own opiates to replace those formerly introduced from the outside. In effect, the brain cannot function normally because some of its neurotransmitters are missing. The addict must experience the agonies of withdrawal until endorphin production returns to normal.

It is not clear whether opiate addiction can cause lasting changes in brain chemistry. One argument that such changes can occur is based on the experience of addicts who are sent to prison, where they are kept away from drugs for years. Some of those individuals will be back on heroin just a few days after their release from prison. Some scientists say that this compulsive drug-seeking behavior is the result of changes in brain chemistry induced by the original addiction. Others maintain that it is caused by social and psychological factors; that is, because former addicts drift back to their old neighborhoods and resume their old ways of life. Neither side has enough evidence to convince the other.

Although explaining drug addiction in terms of endorphins and opiate receptors may seem convincing, it does not tell the whole story about the activity of opiates in the brain. For example, one way to regard drug addiction is as a psychological phenomenon, a *conditioned response*. We all have conditioned responses to things that happen to us. We tend to repeat actions that benefit us and avoid ones that hurt us.

The conditioned response theory of addiction holds that the addict takes heroin both to avoid a negative sensation (namely, the withdrawal symptoms that cause pain when the drug supply is cut off) and to achieve a positive response, or "reward" (the initial rush of euphoria obtained when the drug is taken). In animal studies, neurobiologists such as Michael A. Bozarth and Roy A. Wise of Concordia Univer-

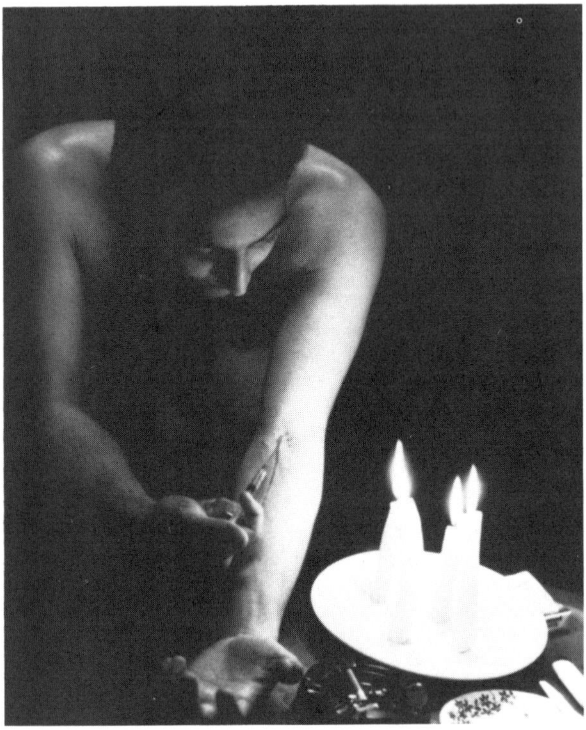

A young addict shooting heroin. Injecting an opiate causes the drug to reach the bloodstream immediately and therefore affect the brain much more rapidly and dramatically than if it had been eaten or smoked.

sity in Montreal have attempted to locate the parts of the brain associated with this two-sided conditioned response to opiates.

In laboratory experiments, Bozarth and Wise have observed that rats learn to press a lever that administers morphine directly into the section of the brain called the *ventral tegmental area.* But injections of morphine directly into this area of the brain do not result in physical dependence; the rats do not show signs of withdrawal symptoms when the injections stop.

Interestingly, the neurotransmitter used by neurons in the ventral tegmental area appears to be dopamine rather than one of the endorphins, which means that two different chemical reactions in the brain might play a role in addiction. One is positive — the one that induces a temporary feeling of euphoria. The other is negative — the one that creates the drive to avoid the agony of withdrawal. The animal experiments indicate that the two mechanisms are associated with different parts of the brain.

Nonaddictive Painkillers

The discovery of the brain's natural opiates has revived hopes for the development of pain-relieving drugs that are nonaddictive. Pharmaceutical companies have investigated synthetic molecules modeled on endorphins, but the results have been disappointing. In animal tests, these synthetic drugs appeared just as addictive as morphine or heroin. The body's own opiates are not addictive because they are swiftly destroyed by enzymes after they act on receptors. Synthetic versions survive for a longer time and therefore cause addiction. But the hope for a nonaddictive pain reliever is still alive. Research shows that, by careful modification of the opiates' molecular structures, it may be possible to disentangle the pain-relieving properties of the drugs from their addictive properties. One relatively nonaddictive artificial opiate, pentazocine (trade name Talwin), is on the market now, and research to develop others continues.

The kinds of studies that solved the opiate mystery have also been conducted on an equally ancient, and in many ways equally dangerous, psychoactive drug — alcohol. But that story is much more complicated, as we shall now see.

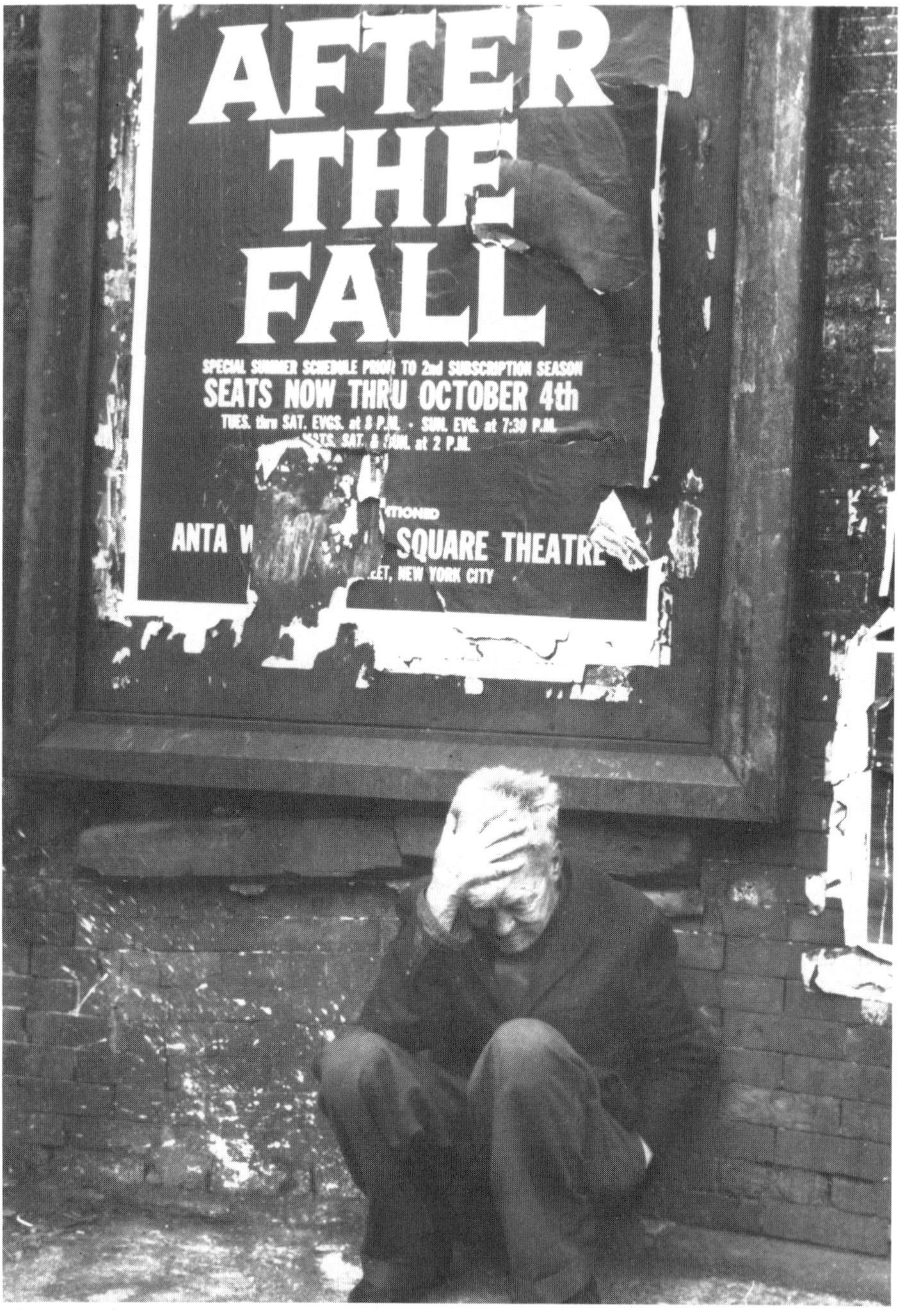

A portrait of alcoholism vividly captures the full ravages of this disease. Chronic drinking can cause damage to neurons in the brain and the deterioration of both mental and physical capabilities.

CHAPTER 3

ALCOHOL AND THE BRAIN

Although alcohol has been a companion of the human race for thousands of years, it is only in the past few decades that it has been considered a drug. Alcohol was traditionally regarded as a kind of food — a food whose abuse could lead to serious physical and mental damage, but a food nonetheless. The work that changed this age-old view of alcohol was done primarily by one researcher, Charles Lieber of Mount Sinai School of Medicine in New York City. Doctors have recorded the debilitating effects of alcoholism for centuries, but they had always attributed the damage not to excess alcohol consumption itself but to other related factors, such as bad diet and poor living conditions. In the late 1960s, working with baboons, Lieber showed that alcohol alone caused the physical damage associated with alcoholism.

Alcohol is now recognized as a *neurotoxin* — a chemical that damages nerves. Not all the damage suffered by alcoholics is caused by alcohol's neurotoxic effects; for example, the most severe brain condition found in chronic alcoholics is related to a vitamin deficiency. But chronic, excess consumption of alcohol is enough to harm the neurons of the brain. *Fetal alcohol syndrome*, a condition found in babies born to mothers who drink excessively during pregnancy, is just one example of alcohol's harmful effects on the brain. Alcohol passes through the placenta (an organ inside the uterus that nourishes the fetus) and interferes with the normal process of brain development. Babies born with fetal alcohol syndrome have abnormally small heads. Their brain size is smaller than normal, and they often suffer some degree of permanent mental retardation.

Used carefully and in moderation, alcohol will not damage the health of most people. Indeed, according to some studies, moderate drinking may lead to a longer life for some people by reducing their chances of suffering a heart attack. When alcohol is consumed in excess, however, it is a deadly drug of abuse. Chronic drinking can lead to physical addiction, involving tolerance and physical dependence. The withdrawal symptoms of alcoholism are well known as ***delirium tremens***, or DTs, characterized by hallucinations, mental confusion, trembling, convulsions, nausea, and irritability. We recognize tolerance when we say that a heavy drinker can "hold his liquor," meaning that the drinker appears sober after consuming enough alcohol to fell a novice. But tolerance only occurs up to a point with alcohol. Chronic alcoholics can become drunk if they take only a small amount of alcohol.

Blood Alcohol Content

Many people think of alcohol as a stimulant, something that will "pep you up," but it is actually a depressant. We feel stimulated when we drink because alcohol loosens the control exercised by higher brain centers. The short-term effects of alcohol consumption — how someone feels and acts after having a few drinks, or a few too many — can be documented fairly precisely in terms of the alcohol content of the blood.

Blood alcohol content, it should be noted, is determined by several factors: quantity of alcohol consumed; whether there is food in the stomach to slow the rate at which alcohol reaches the blood; and even the body size of the drinker (a bigger person will have a lower blood alcohol concentration than a smaller individual who drinks the same amount because there is more body tissue to absorb the alcohol).

A drinker begins to feel loose and less inhibited when the level of alcohol in the blood reaches 0.05%. Alcohol achieves its behavioral effects by working on the *reticular activating system*, a part of the brain that plays a role in controlling the flow of information from all the sensory systems of the body to the cerebral cortex, which is the center of higher thought processes.

When blood alcohol concentration reaches 0.1% the drinker is overtly clumsy, and reaction time to a visual stimulus or a sound is slower than normal. The laws of most states set the legal limit for blood alcohol content at 0.1%. Anything higher is defined as drunkenness.

The danger inherent in drinking and driving is that even moderate levels of blood alcohol produce a treacherous and seductive set of conditions. The drinker relaxes and often develops a false sense of confidence. The feeling is deceptive. Intoxication is accompanied by a tendency to underestimate the speed of moving objects and a loss of coordination. Coupled with a delusion of heightened competence, the neurological impairment caused by alcohol can be disastrous.

As blood alcohol content increases above 0.1%, more brain control centers are progressively affected. At a blood level of 0.2%, the activity of the entire motor area of the brain is significantly depressed. The drinker is staggering and uncoordinated — or perhaps lying down. The emotional control centers, such as the limbic system, are also out of whack, with unpredictable results. Some drinkers become angry, others become sad and weepy, sometimes expressing at the top of their lungs feelings that are usually kept under control.

A woodcut depicts a man afflicted with delirium tremens (DTs), a term describing the symptoms of alcohol withdrawal. DTs are characterized by hallucinations, mental confusion, and physical disorders such as trembling, convulsions, and nausea.

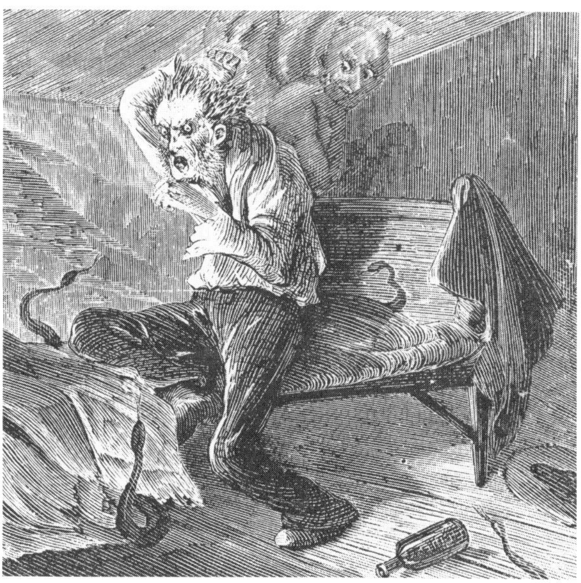

Effects become even more serious at higher blood alcohol levels. At 0.3%, the drinker is hopelessly confused and may fall into a stupor. A blood alcohol content of 0.4% causes coma, and a level of 0.5% depresses the *medulla oblongata*, the part of the brain stem that controls breathing, enough to cause death by respiratory failure in two or three hours. (Lower blood alcohol levels, in the neighborhood of 0.4%, can be fatal if they hit the body suddenly, as when a drinker belts down a bottle of whiskey in a few minutes.)

Long-term Effects of Alcohol

The long-term effects of alcohol consumption have also been studied intensively. Alcohol is different from other psychoactive drugs because it can cause visible anatomical changes in the brain that are easily detected in a number of ways. One effect of chronic alcoholism is a decrease in brain size. Shrinkage of the brain caused by atrophy, or wasting away, of the brain cells has been measured in many alcoholics. In the past, this shrinkage was found during autopsies. Today, the effects of chronic drinking on the living brain can be measured by such advanced techniques as computerized tomography (CT) scans, which give X-ray pictures of brain structure.

Shrinkage can easily be seen in CT images. One measure of shrinkage is the size of the *ventricles*, the fluid-filled cavities in the central part of the brain under the cerebral cortex. Several studies have noted an increase in ventricle size in chronic alcoholics, who in effect have less brain and more empty space. Another measure of brain atrophy is the size of the *sulci*, the valleys on the surface of the cortex. Wider sulci are an indication of brain atrophy; they are often found in the brains of individuals suffering from senility or alcoholism.

A series of CT scans done on confirmed drinkers has produced evidence that chronic alcoholism causes progressive shrinkage of the brain. Most of those studies show only minor widening of the ventricles and the sulci in younger alcoholics. The amount of widening — and hence the amount of brain atrophy — tends to be greater in older alcoholics, in proportion to the severity of the alcoholism.

A result of brain atrophy is the loss of some mental capabilities. The loss is selective. Studies of hundreds of alcoholics have found that they perform close to normal in tests of often-repeated verbal skills, such as vocabulary and word comprehension. But alcoholics suffer losses in nonverbal skills — the ability to solve problems involving shapes and space, to reason abstractly, and to perform physical tasks requiring careful hand-eye coordination.

In one such test an individual is shown a number matched with a symbol. Later, the individual is given the number and must draw the symbol. Other tests measure the ability to assemble several parts into a complete object and to reproduce a design using colored blocks. Alcoholics consistently perform poorly on these tests. They also do poorly on tests of memory.

Alcohol itself is only secondarily responsible for some of these effects. Alcoholics have poor eating habits and resultant vitamin deficiencies; they are vulnerable to a number of diseases; they often suffer head injuries in repeated falls. Some experts also believe that there is an underlying brain abnormality in some people that leads them to become alcoholics in the first place and that shows up on mental tests. Yet there is evidence that alcohol in itself does contribute to brain damage. Among other things, studies have found that social drinkers have memory losses of the same kind, but milder, than those experienced by alcoholics, and that the losses appear to be related to the amount of alcohol consumed; occasional drinkers are less affected than people who drink frequently.

At the far end of the spectrum is the most severe kind of alcoholic brain damage, called the *Wernicke-Korsakoff syndrome*, which occurs in extreme cases of long-term, chronic alcoholism. One part of the syndrome is a set of neurological symptoms that includes overall confusion, visual problems, loss of muscle coordination, and general nerve damage. Treatment with large doses of thiamine, a vitamin, can reverse some of these symptoms. Without thiamine treatment, the patient may die. Although a shortage of thiamine — a dietary problem — is obviously a cause of Wernicke-Korsakoff syndrome, nerve damage by alcohol is believed to be at least partly responsible.

Wernicke-Korsakoff syndrome can also cause amnesia, striking personality changes, and a compulsion to recite imaginary experiences, perhaps in an effort to fill in memory gaps. Wernicke-Korsakoff patients are usually passive, apathetic,

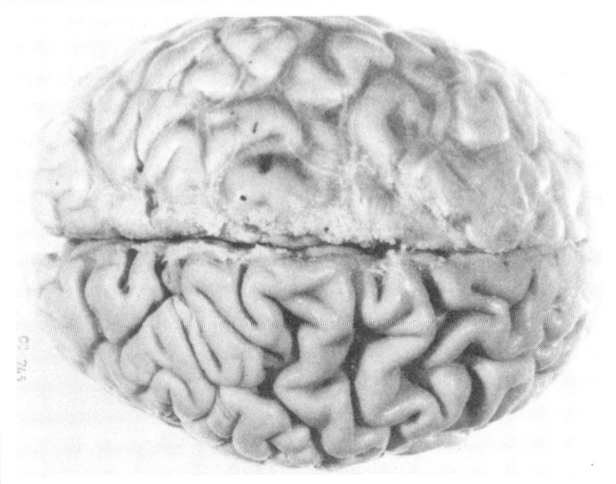

A photograph showing the brain of an alcoholic who suffered from brain atrophy. This condition is characterized by widened valleys, or sulci, on the surface of the cerebral cortex. Brain atrophy is a chief consequence of chronic alcoholism and leads to the loss of mental capabilities.

and indifferent to the world around them. Most must be institutionalized for life.

Except in such extreme cases, it appears that many of the effects of chronic drinking on the brain can be reversed if the drinker gives up alcohol. A series of CT scans of the brains of chronic alcoholics has shown that brain size begins to increase when drinking stops. Both the ventricles and the sulci grow smaller as the brain grows larger. At the same time, tests of performance show improvement. Verbal abilities appear to show the fastest recovery, with sensory and motor function not far behind. More complex abilities, such as short-term memory, visual spatial learning, and abstract thinking, improve at slower rates. Yet, even years after they give up drinking, former alcoholics still have some brain deficits.

Where in the Brain Does Alcohol Strike?

Neuroscientists still cannot agree on the exact brain structures and functions that are damaged by chronic alcohol abuse. One theory is that alcohol causes generalized brain damage, but critics of the theory point out that not all brain functions suffer equal losses.

Another theory is that alcohol damages the limbic system and the right front lobe of the cerebral cortex, which governs perceptual and spatial skills. The theory proposes that verbal abilities, which are controlled by the left side of the cortex, suffer less because they are in more constant use. Those who support this theory point out that people who suffer non-alcohol-related damage to the right side of the cortex have many of the problems reported in chronic alcoholics.

A third theory is that alcohol damages the region of the brain that transmits messages from the front part of the cerebral cortex. This hypothesis is supported by studies showing decreased blood flow in that part of the brain in alcoholics. But none of the theories has enough evidence behind it to convince all scientists studying the brain.

Another issue that remains in doubt is whether social drinkers suffer a loss of intellectual abilities similar to what alcoholics experience but less severe in nature. There is some evidence to indicate that they do and that the critical factor is the total amount consumed at one time. A study done by Dr. Elizabeth Parker questioned 1,365 men and women about their drinking habits and had them take tests of intellectual performance. There was a relationship between decreased performance on a test that required the ability to relate different ideas and the amount of alcohol consumed during a typical drinking occasion. In some studies, memory losses have also been detected in social drinkers, and the amount of loss seems to be related to the amount of alcohol consumed. All the evidence is not in yet, but it does appear that steady drinking can cause impaired brain function over a period of years.

What can be called the gross effects of alcohol — brain shrinkage and a loss of mental function — have been studied for many years. The question of how alcohol acts on a molecular level to affect brain cells is much newer. It also has a surprisingly complicated answer. In the previous chapter, we saw that the effects of morphine and heroin can be explained by the existence of natural opiates in the body. It is not that simple with alcohol. To understand how alcohol acts, we must also look at two other categories of psychoactive drugs—the barbiturates and the tranquilizers.

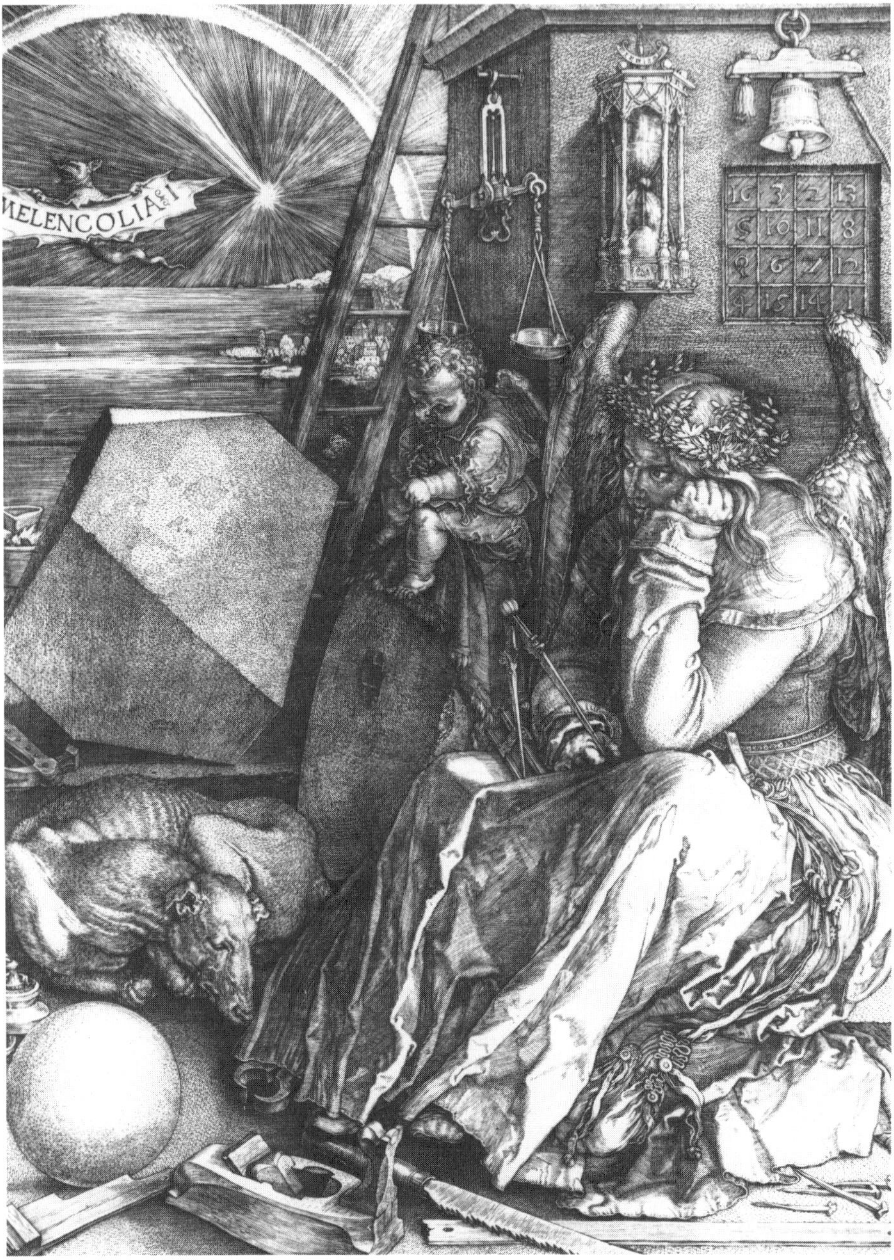

Albrecht Dürer's 1514 engraving Melancholia *depicts the condition most of us know as depression. Barbiturates, tranquilizers, and alcohol are all central nervous system depressants and can cause downward mood changes even when consumed in moderate amounts.*

CHAPTER 4

BARBITURATES, TRANQUILIZERS, AND ALCOHOL

We do not often think of alcohol as a tranquilizing drug. We do not often think of anxiety as a disease. Yet there is a great deal of truth to both descriptions. One of the most common reasons for having a drink is to relax after a busy day or an anxiety-provoking encounter. Although anxiety is a normal part of life, for some people it can be an overwhelming burden. All of us feel anxiety when we face a challenge. A few of us feel anxiety all the time — to such an extent that even everyday events become an impossible challenge.

Anxiety and Drug Therapies

At least one in every twenty Americans is estimated to suffer from anxiety severe enough to require treatment. Untreated, anxiety can lead to crippling depression. These people suffer from an exaggerated version of a normal response to the world around them. Fear is nature's way of alerting the body in a dangerous situation. *Hormones* (products of living cells that stimulate other cells) flow through the blood to increase the heart's output of blood and the body's oxygen supply, to tighten the muscles, and to alert us in a number of ways.

The problem arises when someone has this reaction when no danger is present. Severe anxiety can cause symptoms resembling those of a heart attack: dizziness, profuse perspiration, a jittery stomach, and blurred vision.

Psychotherapy has been able to help some patients suffering severe anxiety, but the mainstay of treatment has been drugs. The original antianxiety drugs were ***barbiturates***, the first of which, barbital, appeared at the turn of the century. Thousands of different types of barbiturates have been developed in the laboratory, and more than a dozen are on the market (although their use has declined steeply in recent years).

If we look at alcohol and the barbiturates carefully, we can see that they have many things in common. Principally, both are sedatives. Indeed, the original reason for using barbiturates to treat anxiety was to calm the disturbed person through mild sedation. Someone who is sleepy and relaxed is less likely to feel the sharp edge of anxiety.

As it turns out, barbiturates are not particularly effective in the treatment of anxiety. Some of them act quickly, putting the patient to sleep in a matter of minutes and keeping him or her sedated for a few hours. Phenobarbital, which is, on the other hand, only moderately sedative and relatively long-lasting, used to be the most popular barbiturate for treating anxiety. But it, too, has severe limitations. Like all the barbiturates, it is addictive. In addition, it has a relatively small safety margin. Barbiturates act on the brain centers that control breathing. The lethal dose — the amount that depresses the breathing center so much that death occurs — is only a few times the amount that causes sedation. For those reasons, barbiturates were usually prescribed only for short periods, when patients were suffering from acute attacks of anxiety or stress.

Tranquilization

The first drug developed to act specifically against anxiety was meprobamate, which was discovered by accident. In the late 1940s Frank Berger, a Czech working in London, was screening compounds more or less at random in an effort to find new antibiotics. When he injected one compound into mice, he saw that they became paralyzed — apparently because they could not use their muscles or limbs — but remained otherwise alert. Berger realized that a muscle-relaxing drug could be used to help human patients with such conditions as back pain. Doctors now prescribe mephenesin, a

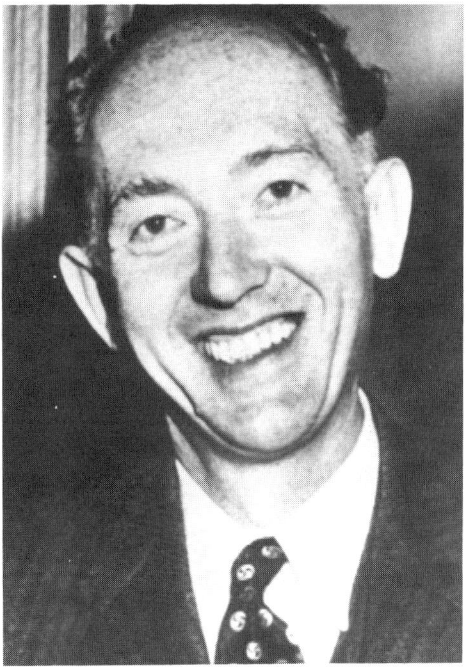

In an effort to develop new antibiotics, the Czech scientist Frank Berger accidentally discovered the drug meprobamate, better known by its trade name, Miltown. Although a potent tranquilizer, Miltown unfortunately proved to be dangerously addictive.

relative of the compound that first produced the effect in mice; this drug is still used medically as a muscle relaxant.

When mephenesin was tested in patients suffering muscle spasms, it appeared to ease their anxiety without making them sleepy — a trait that Berger had noted in animal experiments and that he called "tranquilization." Meprobamate was a molecular derivative of mephenesin that Berger discovered in the course of a methodical series of tests to find an effective human tranquilizer.

Meprobamate was put on the market in the United States under the trade name Miltown in 1955 and was an immediate success. Berger seemed to have found a compound that acted directly on the brain centers that cause anxiety. It appeared not only to offer the antianxiety effects of phenobarbital without sedating the patient, but also to be nonaddicting.

The first impression changed drastically as more tests of meprobamate's effects were conducted. Studies found few differences in the effects that meprobamate and phenobarbital had on brain activity; both caused about the same level of drowsiness. And meprobamate was found to be addicting.

Taken over time, it caused both tolerance and physical dependence. Patients who stopped taking meprobamate suddenly experienced hyperactivity, anxiety, and, sometimes, convulsions.

The Birth of a Billion-Dollar Business

But the early reports on meprobamate stimulated a search for other compounds that could relieve anxiety without causing sedation. In many respects it was not a sophisticated search. Some drug companies simply tested compounds at random, because they had no idea how meprobamate produced its effects. Success came completely by accident in the laboratory of Leo Sternbach, a chemist at what was then the Roche Drug Company.

Sternbach was working with a family of newly synthesized chemicals called *quinazolines*, most of which had no effect on laboratory animals. Many months after he gave up the work, Sternbach found what he thought was one last quinazoline stored away in a corner of his laboratory and gave it to his boss for testing. It turned out to have a highly tranquilizing effect in animal tests. When the chemical was analyzed, it was discovered not to be a quinazoline at all, but rather a member of a family of compounds that is now called the *benzodiazepines*. Thus was Valium, on which a billion dollar business is based, discovered.

The first benzodiazepine was marketed as an antianxiety drug in 1960 under the trade name Librium. A close relative was put on the market three years later. Its generic name is diazepam; it was marketed as Valium. In terms of sales, both are among the most successful drugs in history; indeed, they were too successful, being prescribed almost routinely for a range of emotional problems that might have been better treated nonchemically. In the mid-1970s, one out of every seven Americans was taking Librium or Valium, and over a hundred million prescriptions a year were being written for them. After repeated warnings of overuse, prescriptions for Librium and Valium dropped, by the mid-1980s, to about one-third of the peak level.

The benzodiazepines are still widely used because they relieve anxiety and are much less sedating and dangerous than barbiturates. A patient who takes a benzodiazepine might experience some drowsiness at first, but that reaction generally wears off after he or she has been taking the drug for a few weeks. It is true that both Librium and Valium can be addicting. Tolerance can develop in time, and drug dependence can develop rather quickly. But the withdrawal symptoms of both are less severe than with other addictive drugs and can be treated more easily. On the positive side, the benzodiazepines are comparatively safe drugs. For example, though it is possible to commit suicide with an overdose of benzodiazepine, it is not easy. Librium and Valium often show up in emergency room accounts of overdoses, but usually in combination with other substances, such as alcohol or a barbiturate.

Cross-tolerance and Cross-dependence

Scientifically, the effect of these combinations offers a fascinating clue to how all these drugs act in the brain. Benzodiazepines potentiate (strengthen) the sedating effects of alcohol and barbiturates, as well as their depressant effects on important brain centers, notably the center that controls breathing. All three kinds of drugs display what is called cross-tolerance, meaning that a patient who develops a tolerance for one of them will show tolerance to the other two. For example, someone who develops tolerance to meprobamate will need larger than normal doses of Valium for the same treatment of anxiety, and vice versa.

All three kinds of drugs also display cross-dependence, meaning that one can be substituted for another in treating cases of drug dependence. For example, benzodiazepines are often used to relieve the symptoms of barbiturate addiction. They are also used to treat delirium tremens, the withdrawal symptoms of alcoholism.

Cross-tolerance and cross-dependence indicate that barbiturates, meprobamate, benzodiazepines, and alcohol all act on the same synapses (nerve endings) in the brain. Yet the evidence indicates that benzodiazepines act at a slightly different site from the other three. Librium and Valium are only mildly sedating. Much larger doses than those prescribed to relieve anxiety are needed to put a patient to sleep. By contrast, the other three kinds of drugs put people and animals to sleep at doses only slightly higher than those needed to treat anxiety.

Barbiturates, Tranquilizers, and GABA

Using opiates as a model, we might expect to find not only receptors for these depressant drugs but also natural versions of the antianxiety drugs in the human body. There are such receptors, but research has failed to find any natural antianxiety molecules in the brain. Instead, neuroscientists have outlined a much more complicated scheme of interactions that involves not only these sedatives but also antianxiety drugs, compounds that cause convulsions, and one neurotransmitter, GABA.

GABA is an inhibitory neurotransmitter and therefore slows the rate at which nerve cells fire. In the early 1960s neuroscientists showed that the inhibitory effects of GABA were increased by alcohol, barbiturates, meprobamate, and benzodiazepines. When laboratory cats were given any of these drugs, the amount of GABA needed to inhibit the firing of specific nerve cells decreased.

A major advance in understanding this interaction came in 1977, when benzodiazepine receptors in the brain were discovered by two research teams, one at the Roche Drug Company in Switzerland and one at Ferrosan, a small Danish drug company. (Pharmaceutical companies invest heavily in this kind of research because of the enormous market potential of psychoactive drugs.) Both used the same method — attaching radioactive tags to Valium molecules and then measuring radioactivity to determine where the molecules could be found on brain-cell membranes. The researchers then tested a large number of benzodiazepine drugs to see how well they competed with the Valium for the receptor sites. They found that the extent to which a given drug bound to the receptors was closely related to that drug's ability to reduce anxiety in human patients. The conclusion was that the receptors were the specific sites of benzodiazepine action in the brain.

Many of these receptors are in the limbic system. Specifically, a high concentration of benzodiazepine receptors is found in the *amygdala*, a part of the limbic system that animal studies have found to be associated with, among other things, control of anxiety. Benzodiazepine receptors are also found at a number of sites in the cerebral cortex. It is believed that the benzodiazepines have their antianxiety action in sites

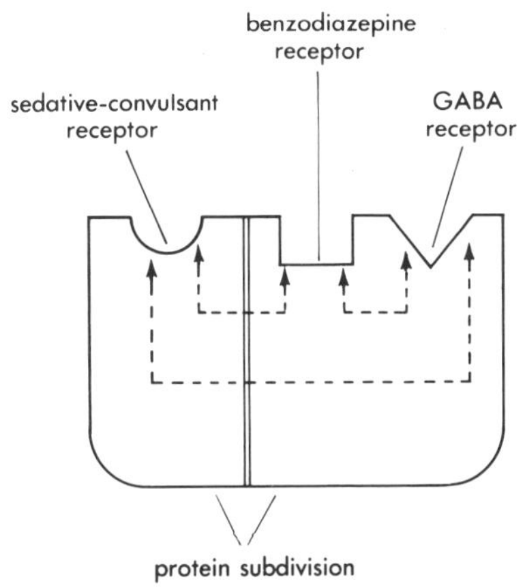

One large protein molecule in neurons contains three different receptors: one for GABA, one for benzodiazepines, and one for both sedatives and convulsants. The location of these receptors on a single molecule enables these chemicals to magnify each other's effects.

located in the limbic system and their sedating action in sites located in the cerebral cortex.

The belief that benzodiazepines act specifically on brain centers that control anxiety has been supported by experiments with drugs called *carbolines*, which have the unusual effect of causing anxiety. Human volunteers who take carbolines experience anxiety far more severe than even that which neurotic patients report. Carbolines are known to bind to benzodiazepine receptors in the brain, a strong indication that the brain centers containing those receptors are part of a natural system regulating anxiety and emotional states.

But as was mentioned, no Valium-like molecules similar to the body's own opiates have yet been found in the brain. Instead, it appears that the benzodiazepines produce their effect through an interaction with GABA. One of the most important steps in this research was taken by John Tallman of the National Institutes of Health. In a series of experiments during the 1970s, Tallman showed that GABA stimulates the binding of Valium to its own receptors. Other researchers then found that Valium, in turn, stimulates the binding of GABA to its own receptors. The explanation was that GABA and benzodiazepines do not occupy the same receptors. Instead, they occupy different receptors that are close neighbors. When GABA binds, it changes the shape of the neighboring receptors so that benzodiazepines bind more efficiently, and vice versa.

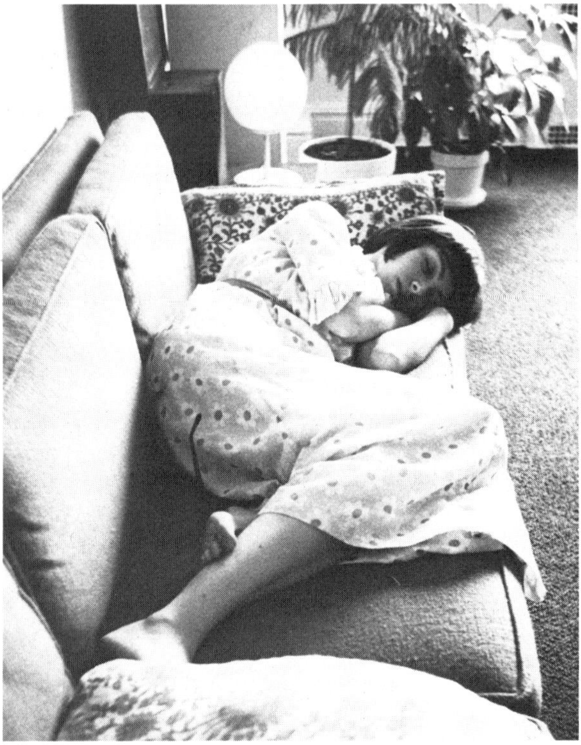

People who use prescription barbiturates to help them sleep must regulate their intake. Not only are barbiturates potentially addictive, but they can be fatal if taken in combination with another drug, such as alcohol.

Neuroscientists have isolated from nerve-cell membranes the large protein molecule that contains both the GABA and benzodiazepine receptors. The same large molecule is also the site of receptors not only for sedatives, including barbiturates and alcohol, but also for drugs that cause convulsions.

The presence of receptors for convulsant drugs on this molecule explains another activity of barbiturates—their ability to block convulsions. (Phenobarbital is often prescribed to control the symptoms of epilepsy.) When neuroscientists did experiments with radioactively tagged convulsant drugs and barbiturates, they found that each inhibited the binding of the other to the receptors. The same was true of meprobamate and alcohol—but not of benzodiazepines, which have no effect on the sedative-convulsant receptors. Yet one thing all the drugs had in common was that they accentuated the activity of GABA on nerve cells.

Neuroscientists could picture a single large molecule that had separate receptor sites for GABA, benzodiazepines, and sedatives such as barbiturates, meprobamate, and alcohol, with the sedative receptor also accepting convulsant drugs. They pictured two subsections of the molecule, one containing the sedative-convulsant receptor, the other containing the GABA and benzodiazepine receptors.

Research on how GABA inhibits the firing of nerve cells added one more part to the receptor-containing molecule. Scientists have found that GABA acts by widening the channels in the nerve-cell membrane through which chloride ions enter the cell. A higher concentration of chloride ions changes the electrical charge of the cell, reducing its ability to fire. Research indicates that the effects of a convulsant drug or sedative are related to its effects on the chloride-ion channel — evidence that the same molecule that contains the sedative-convulsant receptor also includes the chloride-ion channel.

In fact, such a molecule has been isolated by Eric Barnard, a neuroscientist at Imperial College in London. It fills the bill exactly, with closely neighboring benzodiazepine and GABA receptors in one section, sedative-convulsant receptors in another, and the chloride-ion channel nearby. Barnard's discovery allows neuroscientists to make exquisitely detailed studies of the interactions among all the substances that act on this one molecule.

For example, scientists now have a reasonably good explanation of why the combination of a barbiturate and alcohol is potentially deadly, and why the same is true of Valium and alcohol. All these drugs act on closely related sites, which means that they could easily increase each other's potency. Neuroscientists have codified many interactions of the drugs that act on this one molecule. They are now doing much more detailed work, including efforts to determine the actual shape of the chloride-ion channel and the precise distance between the GABA and benzodiazepine receptors.

Some basic questions, however, have not yet been answered. Scientists still do not know why benzodiazepines act only to reduce anxiety, whereas barbiturates act as sedatives. An answer to that question could lead to better and safer sedatives and antianxiety drugs.

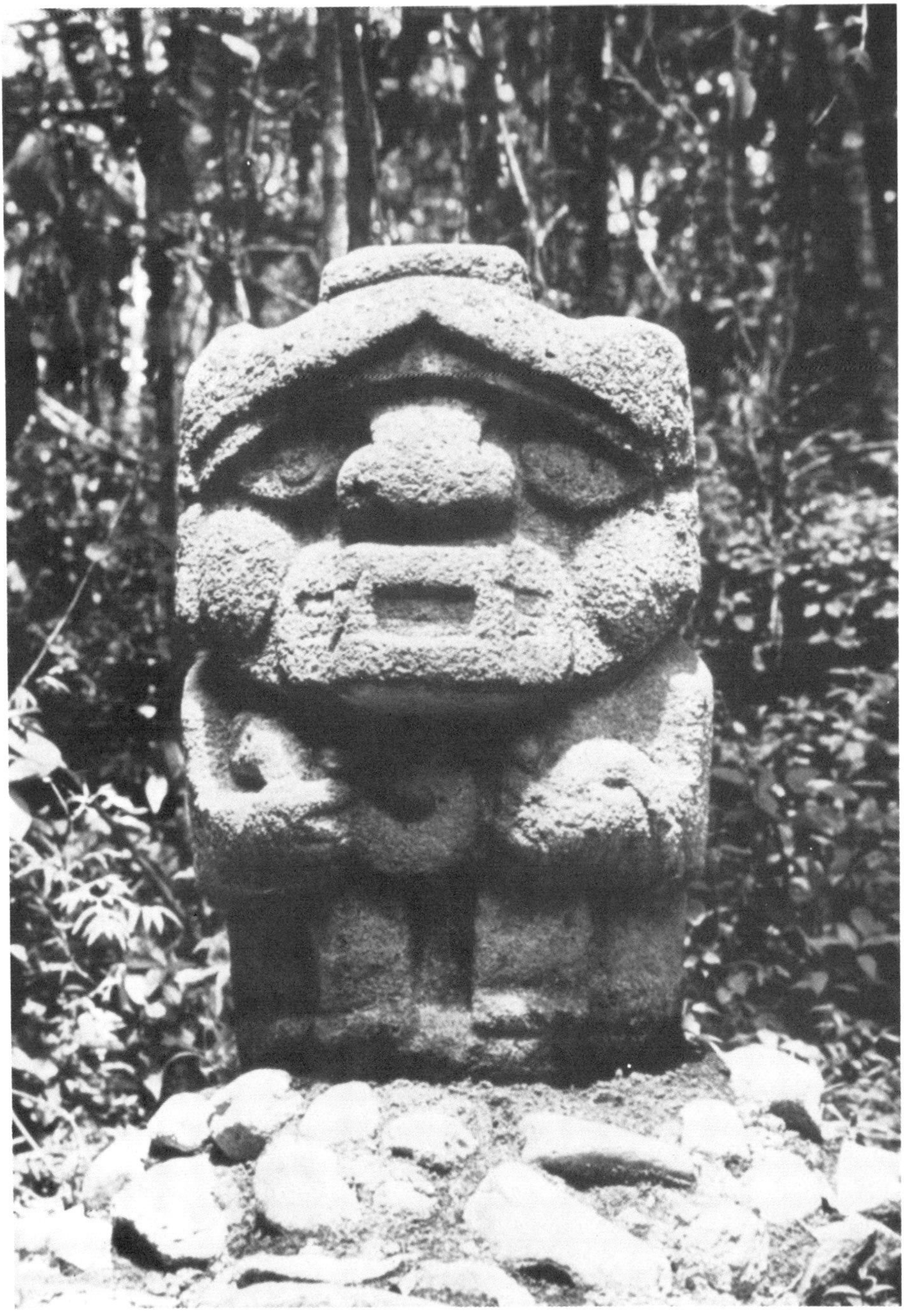

A centuries-old Incan carving portrays a figure chewing coca leaves. The Incas of ancient Peru used coca to increase endurance and appease hunger and to celebrate religious rituals.

CHAPTER 5

STIMULANTS: COCAINE AND THE AMPHETAMINES

Cocaine and amphetamines have vastly different histories, but they have two major things in common. In the short run, they make people feel good and improve alertness and performance. But in the long run (and sometimes in the short run — indeed, in a matter of minutes) they can be enormously destructive. It was the stimulating, "feel good" effects of cocaine and amphetamines that first attracted attention, both in medicine and in street abuse. It took a while to realize that these benefits carried a high price. Sudden death, addiction, brain damage, and a kind of psychosis startlingly similar to *paranoid schizophrenia* (a mental disorder characterized by unwarranted feelings of persecution) are among the potential dangers of cocaine and amphetamine abuse.

When the dangers became evident, the medical uses of both drugs were cut back sharply. Abuse of these drugs, however, did not decrease. Cocaine, once a fairly scarce commodity, is now described as "the drug of the '80s." Amphetamine abuse has been heightened by the appearance of so-called designer drugs such as MDMA, popularly called Ecstasy, which can be produced by simple chemical manipulation of the basic amphetamine structure to produce an even more potent drug.

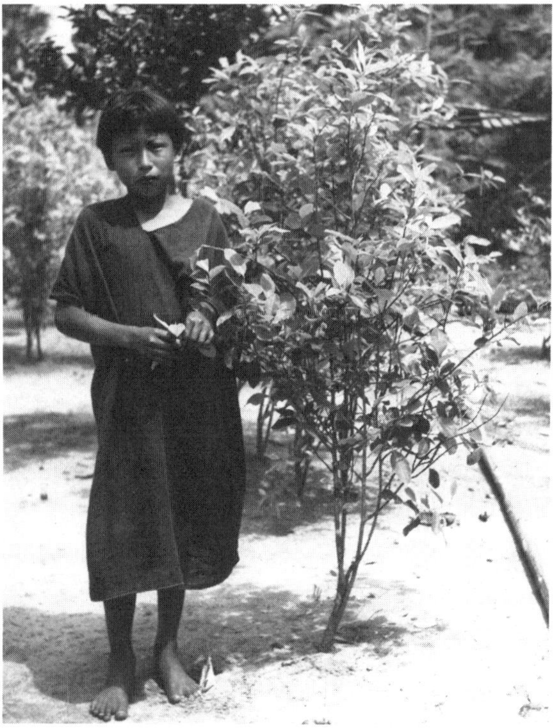

A boy in southern Colombia tends a coca plant. Coca, the plant from which cocaine is derived, is the major cash crop for several South American countries.

The Development of Cocaine

Cocaine has a far longer history than amphetamines. A thousand years ago, South American Indians chewed the leaves of the coca plant to give them more energy for their work. The Spanish brought coca leaves to Europe, where they were used in beverages. In the United States, the original version of Coca-Cola contained a coca-leaf extract; it was eliminated from the drink decades ago, when the dangerous effects of cocaine were discovered.

The medical history of cocaine began with its isolation from the coca leaves in 1860 by Albert Neiman, a German chemist. Its greatest medical proponent was, of all people, the great Viennese psychotherapist Sigmund Freud. As a young neurologist in Vienna, Freud studied cocaine as a treatment for nervous exhaustion. Its ability to improve energy, alertness, and mood greatly impressed him. In 1884 Freud wrote *Über Coca*, a widely read work, in which he claimed that cocaine's apparent benefits could be enjoyed "without any of the unpleasant aftereffects that follow exhilaration brought about by alcohol."

Freud claimed that cocaine could not only cure many diseases and ailments but could also treat narcotic addiction. In fact, he was so convinced of the healing properties of the drug that he prescribed it as treatment for his close friend, Ernst von Fleischl-Marxow, who was addicted to morphine. With tragic irony, Fleischl-Marxow began to use cocaine excessively and subsequently suffered toxic psychosis and died. Freud did not cease his own use of cocaine for many years, but he did begin to write about the newly discovered dangers of the drug.

As more of cocaine's ill effects became evident, it was discredited as a medicine, except for one use that Freud also described: cocaine is an effective anesthetic that can block pain without putting the patient to sleep. Procaine, a drug derived from it, is still used in eye surgery and dentistry.

The Amphetamine Story

The amphetamine story is shorter but more complicated. The first amphetamine was marketed in the 1930s under the brand name Benzedrine as a nonprescription inhalable drug for asthma. Doctors soon reported that students had discovered that Benzedrine increased the feeling of alertness and were swallowing the contents of Benzedrine inhalers to help them cram for final exams.

Amphetamines became immensely popular during World War II. Military leaders were naturally interested in compounds that could improve the mood, alertness, and performance of their troops, apparently without side effects. The armed forces of all major nations took millions of amphetamine tablets during the war. The U.S. armed forces did not give out amphetamines, but American troops often obtained them from the British. The peak use of amphetamines in the U.S. armed forces actually came in the 1960s, when an estimated 225 million pills were taken.

By then, the dangers of amphetamines had become evident. They had emerged as major drugs of abuse, and many serious studies of their effects on the brain were undertaken. Scientists attempted to sort out their valid uses, which turned out to be few. Today, amphetamines are mainly prescribed for two conditions, both of which involve the brain centers concerned with alertness. One condition is *narcolepsy*, which makes patients fall asleep frequently during the day, sometimes even when they are standing up. Amphetamines can counter the tendency to fall asleep, but they do not actually cure narcolepsy, and increasingly larger doses are needed to maintain the effect.

The second therapeutic use of amphetamines is for a childhood behavioral problem called *hyperactivity* (or, more formally, *attention deficit disorder*). Hyperactive children do badly in school because they cannot sit still or pay attention long enough to learn. Their intelligence is usually not affected, but they simply cannot concentrate. It may seem odd to give overactive children a drug that increases activity, but amphetamines are effective against hyperactivity. Apparently, they act on brain centers to increase alertness, allowing the children to concentrate on their tasks.

The most frequent medical use of amphetamines used to be for weight control. Both cocaine and amphetamines act on the appetite centers of the brain to suppress the desire for food, although that effect wears off in a few weeks. Today, amphetamines are prescribed for at most a week or two in weight reduction programs. The stimulating and appetite-reducing effects of amphetamines are clearly two separate activities, because researchers have been able to develop amphetamine derivatives that control appetite but do not stimulate the individual.

Cocaine, Amphetamines, and Mental Disorders

The effects of cocaine and amphetamines on different mental illnesses cast a sharp light on how they act in the brain. To begin with, amphetamines have no beneficial effect on severe depression. In fact, they can make it worse — a surprising finding for drugs that usually produce feelings of euphoria and well-being. When amphetamines are given to patients suffering depression, about half of them experience euphoria for a few hours, while the others feel no effect. Once the temporary euphoria wears off, the underlying depression reasserts itself, often with increased intensity. Interestingly, the patients who experience amphetamine euphoria have the best response to standard antidepressant drugs, an indication that the amphetamines act on some of the brain centers affected by antidepressants.

The long-term effects of either cocaine or amphetamines often include psychosis. Victims of this psychosis know who and where they are, but they also hear voices and experience a steady, growing feeling that the world is conspiring against them. Everything they hear or see seems to be part of this conspiracy, plotted by an army of enemies that fills their world. These delusions can lead to violence, as the addict strikes back at imaginary plotters.

Psychiatrists are familiar with this kind of psychosis in schizophrenic patients who are not drug abusers. The condition is called paranoid schizophrenia, a form of the disease that includes delusions of persecution. Some addicts suffering from stimulant psychosis are diagnosed as having paranoid schizophrenia before psychiatrists learn of their drug abuse.

There are other links between schizophrenia and stimulants. Some schizophrenic patients who are in remission suffer relapses when they take even small doses of amphet-

Many U.S. soldiers in the Vietnam War were given amphetamines to improve their mood and performance. Although the armed forces of other nations routinely took amphetamines during World War II, the U.S. military did not begin this practice until years later.

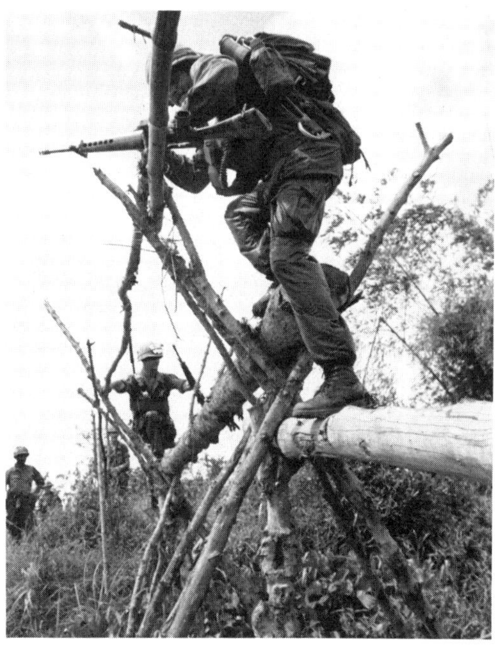

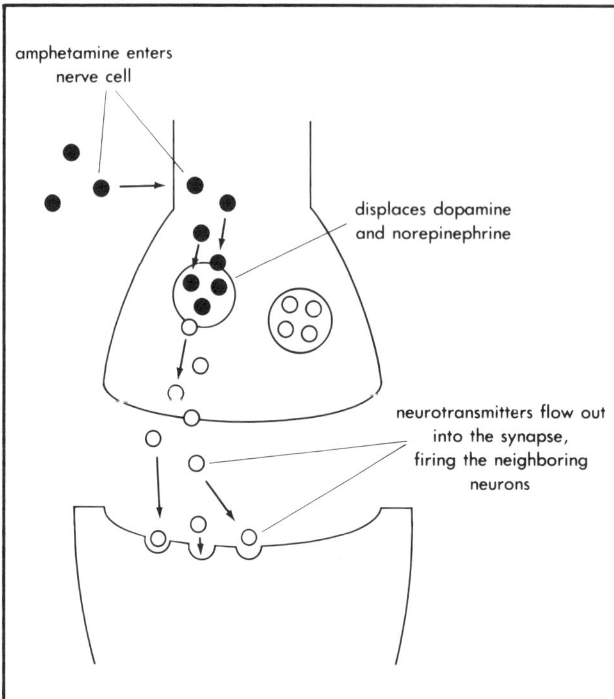

This drawing depicts the action of amphetamine, which produces its stimulating effects by forcing the neurotransmitters dopamine and norepinephrine out of neurons and flooding the nervous system with them.

amines, and the drugs used to treat schizophrenia are the most effective treatments for cocaine and amphetamine psychosis. The effect is so striking that drug companies now test the effectiveness of compounds against schizophrenia by studying how well they block the activity of amphetamines in mice.

Dopamine and Norepinephrine

The resemblance between stimulant psychosis and schizophrenia helps explain how cocaine and amphetamines work on a molecular level. The connecting thread seems to be dopamine and norepinephrine, two neurotransmitters that are catecholamines. Several clues point in the same direction. First, amphetamines have a strong structural resemblance to both catecholamines. Second, drugs that help schizophrenics return to normal behavior appear to act on dopamine pathways. Dopamine neurons help control the limbic system, which regulates emotional behavior. Third, most norepinephrine receptors are found in a small but very important part of the brain stem called the *locus coeruleus. (Coeruleus* is Latin for "blue," and this center is, in fact, blue.)

The locus coeruleus has only a few thousand nerve cells, but their axons run to as many as a third of all the cells of the brain — up to the cerebral cortex, the center of higher thinking; down to the *cerebellum*, the regulation center for fine motor coordination; and out to the spinal cord, where the axons make contact with neurons that regulate muscles of the arms and legs — with many branches along the way. No other center is known to interact with as many parts of the brain. Because of these many connections, the norepinephrine neurons of the locus coeruleus are believed to have something to do with our responses to emotional situations. It is known that these neurons become active during the response to emotion-arousing events, and many neuroscientists believe that this activity helps produce such emotional reactions as a mother's love for her infant or a child's sadness when a toy is broken.

Cocaine and amphetamines produce their stimulating effects by enhancing the activity of norepinephrine and dopamine neurons. It appears that they act in slightly different ways. Neuroscientists have established that amphetamines

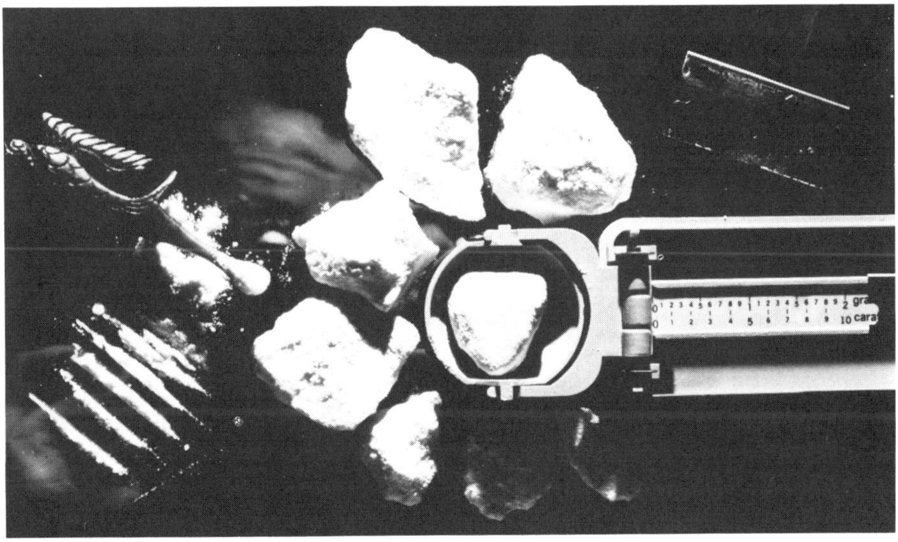

Crack, a particularly addictive and dangerous form of cocaine, is processed into small "rocks" and usually smoked in a pipe. The drug received its nickname because it emits a crackling noise when smoked.

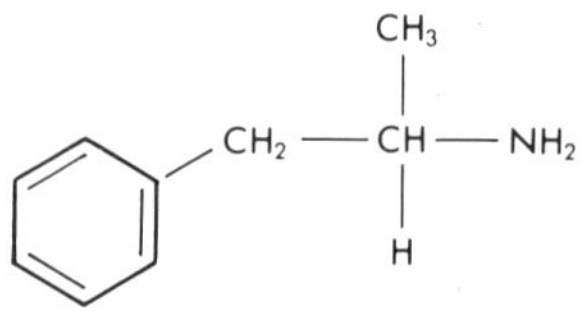

amphetamine

The chemical structure of amphetamine. Chronic users of this stimulant often "hear voices" and suffer delusions of persecution — symptoms identical to paranoid schizophrenia, which is a serious mental disorder.

enter nerve cells and displace dopamine and norepinephrine from their storage sites near the synapses. The neurotransmitters flow out into the synapse, firing the neighboring neurons. Amphetamines also increase activity by interfering with the pump that "sweeps" the neurotransmitters out of the synapse and back into the neurons.

How cocaine acts is not as well understood, although it also appears to interfere with the functioning of dopamine and norepinephrine. The exact action on the molecular level is not clear, but the overall effect on the brain and nervous system centers can be outlined. Cocaine and amphetamines produce a feeling of euphoria by stimulating parts of the limbic system. They make users feel alert by increasing the activity of norepinephrine cells in the higher thought centers of the cerebral cortex. By stimulating norepinephrine cells that regulate motor activity, they give the user the impression — and sometimes the reality — of enhanced muscle strength and endurance.

Cocaine and amphetamine psychosis can also be explained by looking at dopamine. Studies have shown that drugs for schizophrenia act by blocking dopamine receptors. Amphetamines and cocaine enhance dopamine release, which explains why even small doses of amphetamines make the symptoms of schizophrenia worse and eventually bring on these symptoms in drug users who take increasingly large doses. The negative effects of cocaine and amphetamines on society are great, but they have served one useful if unexpected purpose in giving neuroscientists valuable clues about the molecular causes of schizophrenia.

One unfortunate trait of cocaine is the unpredictability of its effects on the brain and other organs. It now appears that cocaine can cause psychosis in some individuals and not others, for reasons that are not fully understood. Cocaine poisoning is equally unpredictable. A cocaine overdose causes convulsions. It can cause death by depressing the brain centers that control breathing and heart activity. Often, death occurs so quickly that treatment cannot help. The well-publicized deaths of several young athletes, the most famous of whom was Len Bias, the University of Maryland basketball player who was the first-round draft choice of the Boston Celtics in 1986, were tragic illustrations of the unpredictability of cocaine poisoning.

Neuroscientists have not detected the same kind of brain shrinkage caused by alcoholism in chronic abusers of cocaine and amphetamines, but there is evidence that the stimulants can cause more subtle brain damage. In animal experiments by Lewis S. Seiden at the University of Chicago, large doses of methylamphetamine were found to reduce the concentration of dopamine in the brain, a sign that there were fewer dopamine neurons. Apparently, methylamphetamine causes neurons to release a massive amount of dopamine, which probably destroys the neurons.

"Designer Drugs"

Experiments with some of the new "designer drugs" derived from amphetamines add evidence to support the view that certain drugs have destructive actions on neurotransmitters. With some relatively simple chemical manipulations, it is possible to produce amphetamine derivatives with different mind-altering qualities. For example, the addition of one chemical group to the methylamphetamine molecule produces MDA (chemical name 3,4-methylenedioxyamphetamine), which not only is a stimulant but also has hallucinogenic effects. Research has shown that at least some of MDA's effects are due to its degenerative action on *serotonin neurons*, which are thought to be involved in mechanisms such as sleep and sensory perception. Studies by Seiden and others at the University of Chicago indicate that MDA has the same degenerative effect on those neurons that methylamphetamine has on dopamine nerve cells.

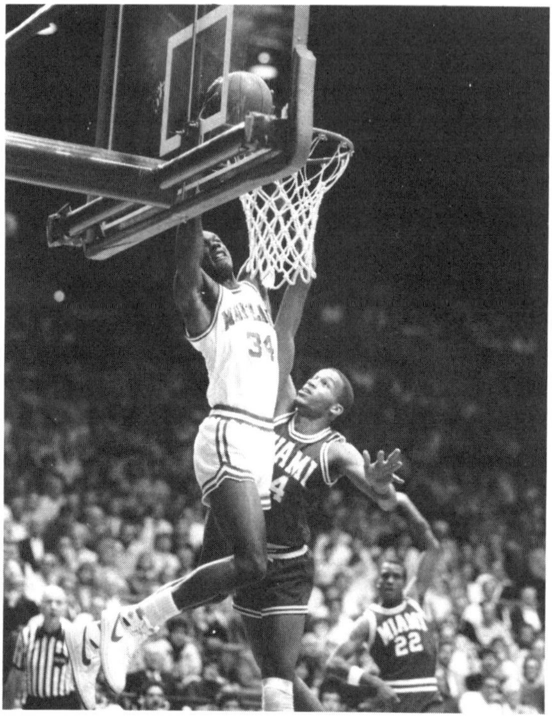

Len Bias, a star basketball player for the University of Maryland, died of a cocaine overdose in 1986. Because a high concentration of cocaine shuts down the brain's control centers for breathing and regulation of heartbeat, an overdose of the drug can cause convulsions, and sometimes death.

A more popular designer drug is MDMA (3,4-methylenedioxymethamphetamine), whose street name is Ecstasy. MDMA was developed in 1914 as a reducing aid, or "diet pill," but was never marketed. It became an increasingly popular street drug in the 1980s and was promoted by some psychiatrists as a help in therapy, on the grounds that it induced an increased sense of awareness but none of the hallucinations and other mental distortions caused by psychedelic drugs — claims that were not supported by clinical research.

Like methylamphetamine, MDMA acts on serotonin neurons. MDMA has not been studied as much as MDA or methylamphetamine, but several animal studies, by Seiden and others, have found evidence of possible damage to serotonin nerve cells. These studies indicate that damage can occur at levels only two or three times higher than the average street dose. MDMA was officially classified as a drug of potential abuse in 1986.

Seiden's studies also provided a possible explanation of the calming effects of MDMA reported by some psychotherapists. In addition to affecting sleep and sensory perception, serotonin neurons play a major role in pain perception and the regulation of aggression and sexual behavior. MDMA probably affects such behavior by depleting the brain's supply of serotonin, Seiden theorized. But because of the evidence that MDMA can destroy serotonin neurons, he warned therapists to test the drug in humans "only with the utmost caution and only if they are convinced that the potential benefits are great enough to outweigh the risks."

However, moves to regulate the use of MDMA cannot prevent the creation and use of other designer drugs. Experience has shown that it is relatively easy to produce molecular variations of many drugs without elaborate laboratories. Experience has also shown that the effects of these drugs are often dangerous and highly unpredictable.

Some of the most beneficial psychoactive drugs have been discovered by accident. The same is true of some of the most damaging drugs. Let us examine some of these accidental discoveries.

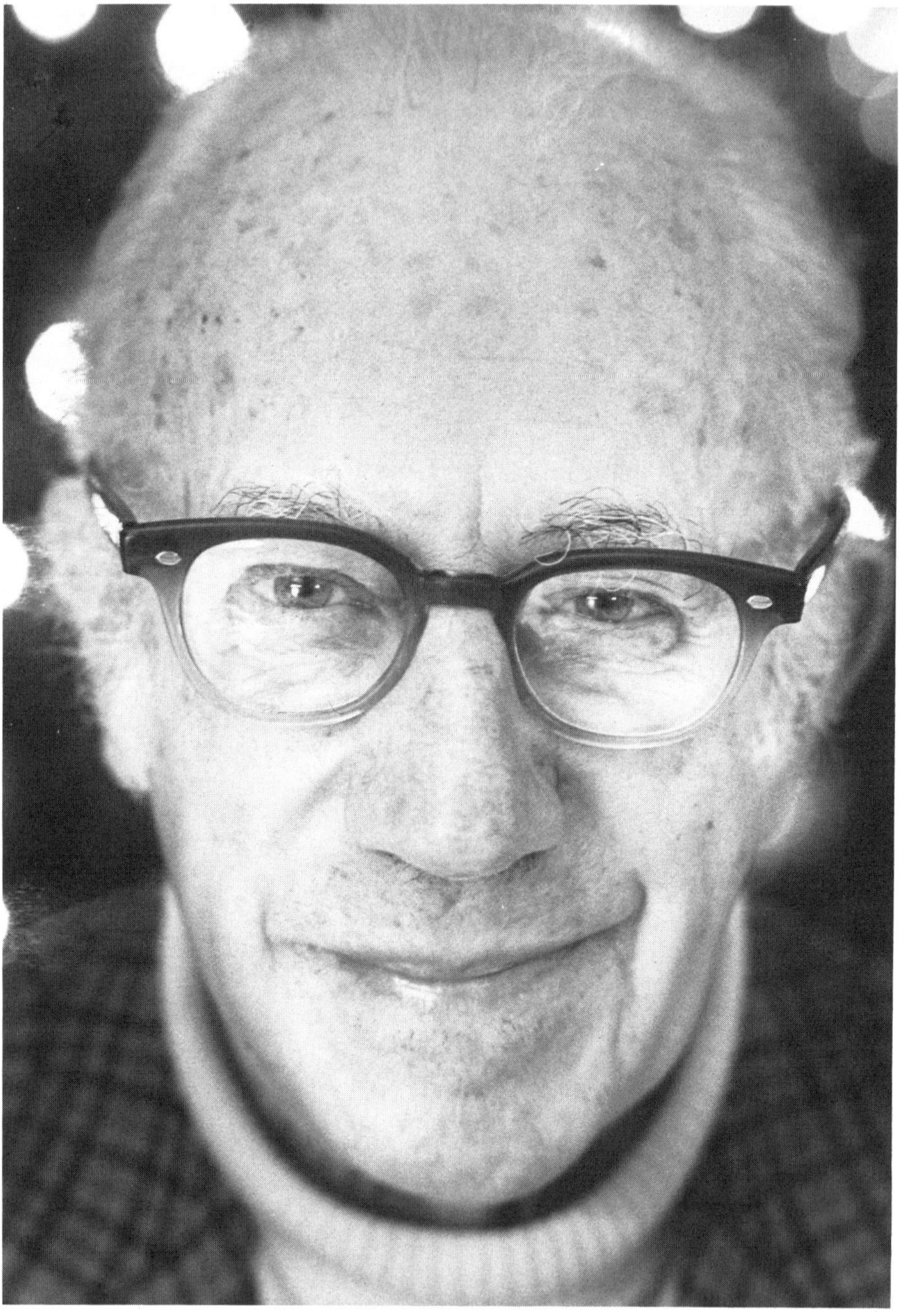

Months after he had given up his attempts to synthesize an effective tranquilizer, Leo Sternbach accidentally created a compound that, in turn, led to the development of the tranquilizer Valium.

CHAPTER 6

ACCIDENTS, GOOD AND BAD

In 1982 doctors at the Santa Clara Valley Medical Center in San Jose, California, began seeing young heroin addicts with an unusual ailment. Despite their youth, they appeared to be suffering from Parkinson's disease, a degenerative nerve disorder that usually afflicts older persons.

The addicts had all the classic symptoms of Parkinson's disease — muscle rigidity; tremor; slow, shuffling movement; even the oily skin peculiar to patients with the disease. The addicts had one thing in common: they had all been using a synthetic heroin produced in an illegal local laboratory. The doctors obtained samples of the drug and had it analyzed. Within months, scientists at Stanford University identified the cause of the problem. The samples contained large amounts of a contaminant, a compound called methylphenyltetrahydropyridine, or MPTP. The MPTP had caused brain damage identical to that found in patients with Parkinson's disease.

Whoever produced the MPTP knew something about drug chemistry, but not enough. The idea was to make a street version of meperidine, a legal narcotic best known by the brand name Demerol. A synthetic version of meperidine appeared on the streets in recent years — MPPP, a compound three times more potent than morphine. If the conditions are not just right, the chemist makes MPTP instead of MPPP.

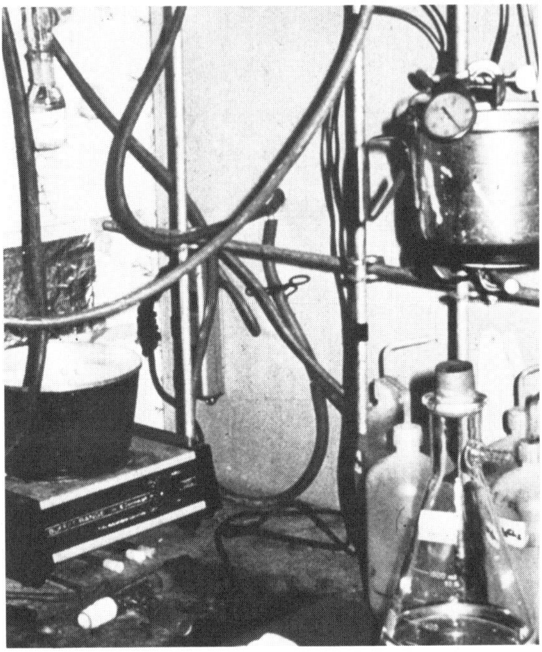

An LSD laboratory. Many of the dangerous "designer drugs" sold on the streets in the 1980s have been synthesized in illegal laboratories. These substances often contain impure toxins.

MPPP was produced legally for some years — and several chemists who worked with it developed symptoms of Parkinson's disease (their samples were contaminated with MPTP). But the link between the contaminant MPTP and the disease was not noted until the addicts came to the hospital in California. For the addicts who took the contaminated drug, the event was a pure disaster. The destruction of the brain cells was permanent, and they were left with symptoms of Parkinson's disease so severe that some of them could barely move. But their tragic experience gave researchers an insight into the possible causes of Parkinsonism.

Neurologists do not know what causes Parkinson's disease in humans, but they do know that autopsies of patients who die of the disease show destruction of neurons in the *substantia nigra*, a brain center that helps control movement. They also know that the concentration of dopamine, a neurotransmitter used by cells in the substantia nigra, is reduced in Parkinson's patients. MPTP both destroyed the neurons in the substantia nigra and depleted the brain's supply of dopamine.

But MPTP's action is startlingly selective. The drug does not destroy all dopamine neurons, only those in the substantia nigra. And it does not have the same effect in all species. Rats are not harmed by MPTP, but monkeys and humans are. Researchers are still trying to unravel the MPTP mystery, but some of their questions have been answered.

Research at a number of laboratories showed that MPTP itself does not destroy nerve cells. Instead, MPTP is metabolized into compounds that are toxic to neurons. Several possible toxins produced by MPTP have been identified. The most likely candidate is a compound called MPP. The fascinating part of this work is that these toxins are produced when MPTP is metabolized by an enzyme named *monoamine oxidase* (MAO), which is interesting for many other reasons, as we shall see.

Meanwhile, the MPTP discovery supports a theory about the way Parkinson's disease develops ordinarily. Neurologists know that a certain percentage of cells in the substantia nigra

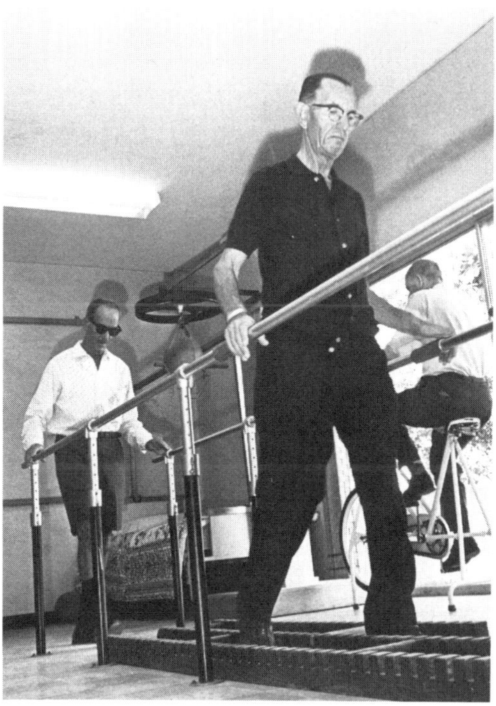

Parkinson's disease patients undergo physical therapy to combat the gradual loss of muscle control that is a consequence of this illness. Scientists have discovered that a drug compound known as MPTP causes brain damage in humans that is strikingly similar to damage found in people suffering from Parkinson's disease.

normally die as a person ages. Parkinson's disease symptoms do not appear until about 80% of the cells have died. So the theory is that most people do not develop Parkinsonism because they retain enough substantia nigra cells throughout their lives. The unlucky ones, the theory proposes, are those exposed to some kind of environmental pollutant that kills enough substantia nigra cells to cause the disease.

No one has yet proved the theory or identified a pollutant that could cause the proposed kind of damage. Neuroscientists are exploring many possibilities. On the more hopeful side, the MPTP discovery has spurred research to develop new drugs that could slow or stop the progressive destruction of brain cells in Parkinson's patients.

As part of the effort to develop drugs to cure Parkinsonism, neuroscientists are trying to establish the exact relationship between monoamine oxidase and MPTP in the brain. Specifically, there are two slightly different versions of monoamine oxidase. Studies indicate that one metabolizes MPTP and the other does not. In animal tests, some drugs that inhibit monoamine oxidase activity have prevented brain damage when MPTP was administered. The hope is to find some version of treatment that might prevent brain damage in humans.

Treating Depression

The discoveries about MPTP and monoamine oxidase illustrate the complexity that neuroscientists face when they study the human brain. For monoamine oxidase is already familiar to them in an entirely different context — the treatment of depression.

When we speak of depression, we refer not to the ordinary low spirits that everyone feels from time to time. We are speaking of depression that afflicts an individual for no identifiable cause and that can be severe enough to incapacitate the sufferer or even lead to suicide. The major event in the modern treatment of depression was the discovery of antidepressant drugs. The first effective antidepressant drug, iproniazid, was introduced in the early 1950s as a treatment for tuberculosis. Its antidepressant activity was discovered through an unlikely chain of events that began with research on drugs for schizophrenia.

A recovering tuberculosis patient monitors her progress in 1952 after taking the drug iproniazid. Introduced in the early 1950s as a treatment for tuberculosis, iproniazid was also found to elevate mood and was eventually prescribed as an antidepressant.

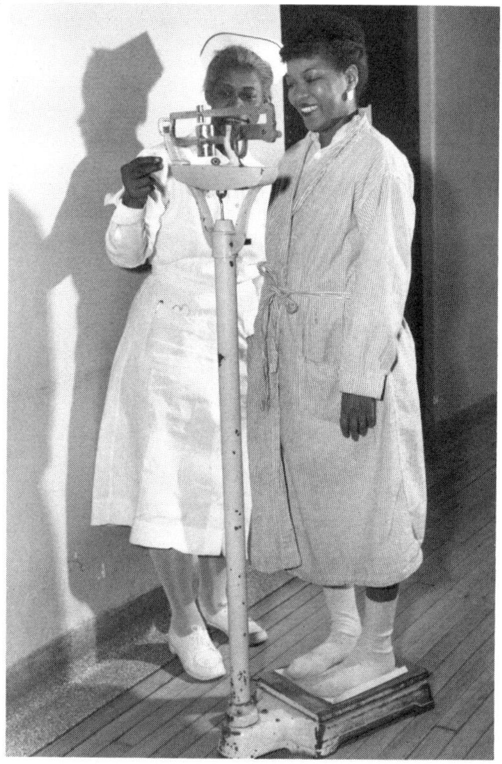

In the 1950s neuroscientists discovered that two drugs, reserpine and chlorpromazine, seemed to be effective in the treatment of schizophrenia. They also knew that reserpine reduced the brain's supply of two chemically related neurotransmitters, norepinephrine and serotonin, which are both classified as amines. (Dopamine is another amine transmitter.) Research showed that when animals were given reserpine, they became sluggish and almost immobile, an effect that some scientists compared to the way the same drug reduced some of the hyperactive behavior shown by schizophrenic patients.

To find other drugs for the treatment of schizophrenia, scientists began screening compounds to see if any would also act on norepinephrine and serotonin. And here monoamine oxidase enters the picture. A biochemist named Albert Zeller had learned that, in the body, amine neurotransmitters are inactivated by monoamine oxidase, an enzyme that removes the amine group from the molecules. Zeller began searching for compounds that would increase the levels of the amine neurotransmitters by inhibiting the activity of monoamine oxidase. He discovered that iproniazid was such a compound.

Monoamine Oxidase Inhibitors

Researchers found that iproniazid reversed the immobilizing effect of reserpine in animals. At the same time, doctors who were using iproniazid to treat tuberculosis reported that patients who took the drug became unusually cheerful. Seizing those clues, a New York psychiatrist named Nathan Kline decided to try iproniazid on depressed patients. It worked, and a new family of drugs was born — the *monoamine oxidase inhibitors*. Researchers soon found a number of compounds that inhibited monoamine oxidase activity. All were effective against depression.

Research showed why. Reserpine depletes the brain's supply of norepinephrine and serotonin by causing them to leak out of the ends of nerve cells. As they leak out, they are inactivated by monoamine oxidase, whose normal function is to scavenge excess neurotransmitter molecules. A compound that stops monoamine oxidase from acting prevents the destruction of the neurotransmitters, which are taken up again by the nerve cells. The end result is increased concentrations of serotonin and norepinephrine in the brain. Somehow, those higher concentrations of amine neurotransmitters relieve the symptoms of depression.

Tricyclic Antidepressants

As they studied monoamine oxidase inhibitors, researchers also stumbled across an entirely different class of antidepressant drugs. Again, the discovery was accidental — a spin-off from the effort to develop new drugs for schizophrenia. Chemists at many drug companies were synthesizing compounds similar to chlorpromazine, then the best available drug for schizophrenia. One of the lookalike compounds that was produced was called imipramine. Tested on schizophrenics, imipramine was a flop. But when imipramine was given to depressed patients (by a doctor who was unable to admit total defeat), they began to improve within several weeks. In a short time, imipramine was on the market as a treatment for depression. It was the first of a new family of drugs, *tricyclic antidepressants*, so called because their chemical structures all contain a three-ring arrangement of molecules.

Then researchers began trying to understand why imipramine worked. Tests showed that imipramine does not inhibit monoamine oxidase activity to any great extent. So the scientists began looking at other ways in which the body might inactivate amine neurotransmitters. A number of studies showed that monoamine oxidase plays only a small part in getting rid of amine neurotransmitters once they have done their work. Monoamine oxidase cleans up after something else has cleared away the majority of the neurotransmitter molecules.

The researcher who did the most to identify the body's main neurotransmitter disposal system was Julius Axelrod, a neuroscientist at the National Institutes of Health. In the 1950s Axelrod began working with neurons from the *sympathetic nervous system*, a division of the autonomic nervous system that regulates such activities as hormone secretion and heartbeat. These nerve cells use norepinephrine as a

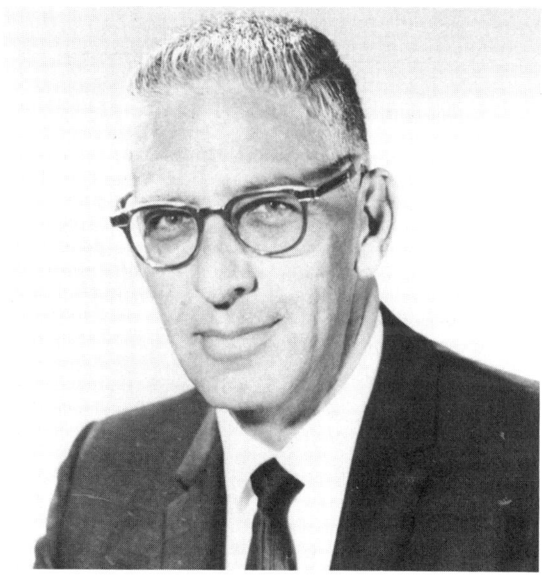

Psychiatrist Nathan Kline won the prestigious Albert Lasker Clinical Research Award in 1964 for his work in identifying the antidepressant properties of iproniazid and related compounds.

neurotransmitter. In a series of studies, Axelrod showed that after norepinephrine molecules transmit a signal, they are pulled back into the neuron that released them by a pumplike mechanism. That was a pivotal finding in neuroscience, because Axelrod had identified the most common disposal system. A few years after he reported his results, other researchers showed that the body rarely uses enzymes such as monoamine oxidase to break up neurotransmitters. Nature is thrifty — instead of breaking up neurotransmitters, the body uses some kind of pumping system to recycle almost all of them. After they transmit a signal, they are pumped back into the neurons for later use.

Taking his research a step further, Axelrod tested the effect of imipramine and other tricyclic antidepressants on the norepinephrine pump. He found that all the drugs interfered with the normal process by which norepinephrine is pumped back into the cells. The drugs increased the amount of amine neurotransmitters, specifically norepinephrine and dopamine, thus increasing the activity of the nerve cells that they affected. It began to seem more and more as if a shortage of those neurotransmitters could cause depression.

Reserpine, Hypertension, and Depression

Several other clues seemed to indicate that neurotransmitters could trigger depression. One was the finding that the limbic system, which regulates emotional behavior, contains many neurons that use norepinephrine and serotonin as neurotransmitters. Another clue came from experience with reserpine in treating high blood pressure, or hypertension. In addition to its effect on schizophrenia, reserpine is highly effective in reducing blood pressure. But the doctors who were using it for that purpose began reporting that even though reserpine was remarkably effective as an antihypertensive, many patients who took it for this purpose were also lapsing into severe depression. Surveys eventually showed that about one of every five patients who takes reserpine develops deep depression — something that seemed clearly related to the depletion of amine neurotransmitters that reserpine causes. In a number of cases, reserpine-related depression is severe enough to result in suicide attempts.

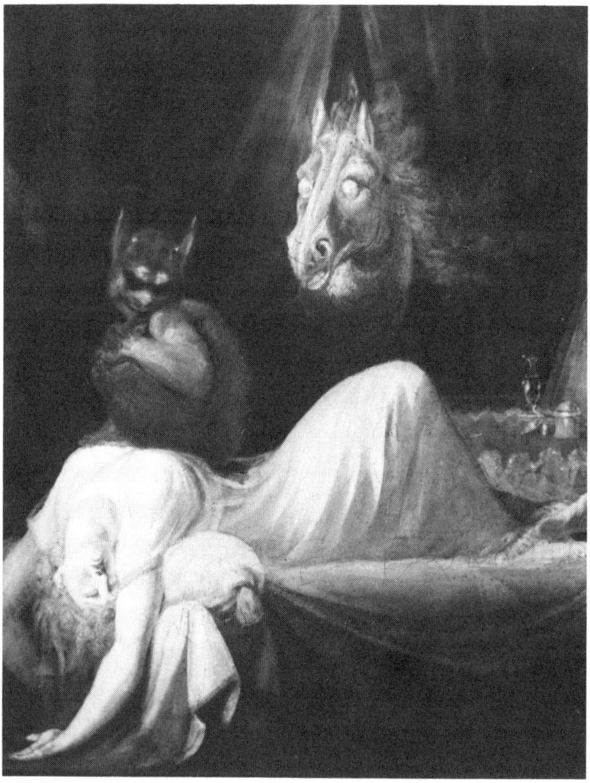

The tormented heroine of Heinrich Fussli's The Nightmare *epitomizes the unspeakable anguish and anxiety that plagues the victims of mental illness. Efforts to ease this sort of suffering have led to many positive breakthroughs in psychiatry and drug research.*

This work has led to the virtual abandonment of reserpine as a drug for the treatment of schizophrenia and high blood pressure alike. It has also led to better treatment for depression. In recent years, a number of new antidepressant drugs that have fewer side effects have been marketed. Neuroscientists do not know exactly how these drugs work, but it is known that they all somehow increase the activity of amine neurotransmitters.

One mystery in the drug treatment of depression is why it takes anywhere from one to four weeks before antidepressants start to show results. The most popular theory is that this time lag has something to do with the brain's normal methods for controlling neurotransmitter levels. According to this theory, neurons that are exposed to increased amounts of neurotransmitters respond by reducing the number of receptors for those neurotransmitters. It is only when the number of receptors stabilizes at a lower level that the increased concentration of neurotransmitters starts to have an effect.

Lithium Carbonate and Manic Depression

Yet another accident, this one based on a misguided theory, led to effective drug treatment for a different kind of depression. Not all people with depression are depressed all the time. Some of them go through cycles in which they swing from deep depression to states of abnormal elation and frantic activity. These emotional swings are the symptoms of a condition known as *manic depression*. During a manic episode, the patient can become overexcited and wildly impulsive, talking endlessly and running off in all directions in pursuit of outlandish schemes. Formerly, the way that doctors could manage these episodes was to put patients to sleep with sedatives and hope they calmed down.

In the 1940s, John Cade, an Australian psychiatrist, developed a theory that manic episodes were caused by some natural toxin in the brain. When he injected the urine of manic patients into animals, Cade thought he detected signs of mania in the animals. Cade wanted to test the effects of uric acid, one of the major waste products in urine, on animals. He could not get the uric acid to dissolve until he mixed it with lithium, a common metal. The combination seemed to calm the animals, and Cade's attention turned to the lithium. He soon was injecting lithium carbonate into manic patients and getting good results.

Cade's toxin theory has been abandoned, but lithium treatment for manic depression has not. It was slow to catch on — first because psychiatrists elsewhere took some time to catch up with the work done by this obscure researcher, second because drug companies were reluctant to market such a low-profit substance — but lithium is now a standard treatment for manic depression. It not only prevents manic episodes but also works against some kinds of depression. Indeed, some patients stop experiencing mania and depression after taking lithium for several years.

To this day, how lithium acts on the brain is unknown. One problem for researchers is that there is no other drug that acts like lithium, so neuroscientists have nothing to compare it with. Another problem is that lithium causes a large number of biochemical changes because of its similarity to sodium, one of the most common chemicals in the blood.

It seems probable that lithium acts on the amine neurotransmitters, but no one has been able to prove that theory yet. A more speculative theory is that there is some kind of chemical seesaw in the brain that keeps emotions under control. In most of us, the seesaw is balanced evenly, so our mood swings are slight. But sometimes the seesaw is unstable. In some people it drops off to the side of depression. In others, it swings from depression to mania and back. If this theory is true, lithium could act in some way to stabilize the chemical seesaw.

It should be noted, however, that depression is not just a matter of chemical imbalance in the brain. Convincing proof that other factors are involved came from a 1986 study that compared antidepressant drug treatment with two kinds of psychotherapy. After a few weeks, the patients taking drugs showed more improvement. But after about four months, drug treatment and psychotherapy produced about the same improvement. Our minds are not just chemical machines.

There are some chemicals, however, that can have a profoundly distorting effect on the way we perceive the world. Let us look at those chemicals now.

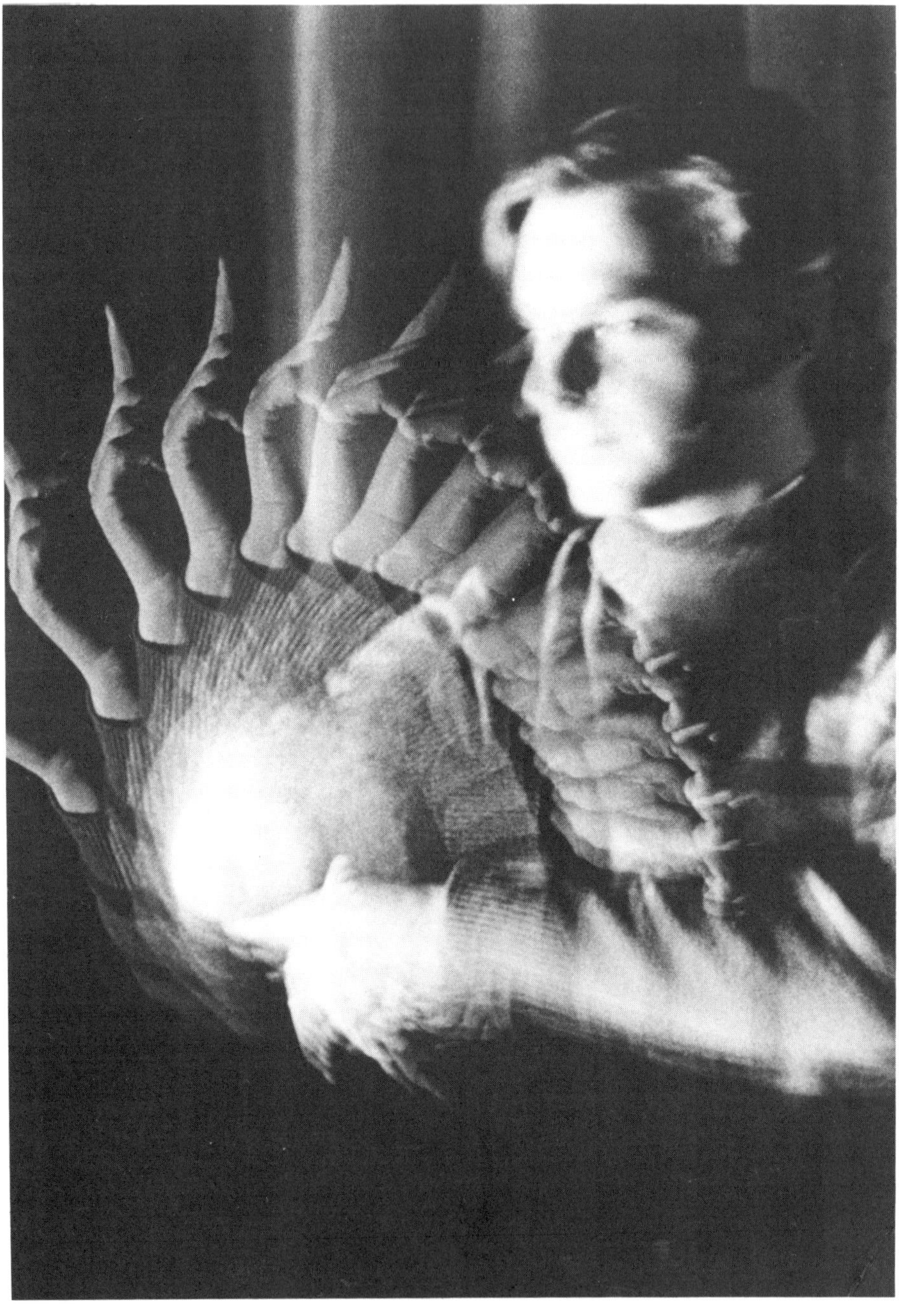

Psychedelic drugs distort perceptions. Users may think that objects are changing shape before their eyes, and they may even believe that sounds can be sensed or "heard" as movements or colors.

CHAPTER 7

PSYCHEDELIC DRUGS

Neuroscientists have learned a lot about the ways that psychoactive drugs act on the brain, but there are still some unanswered questions. At the present state of knowledge, a neuroscientist can often say with certainty which neurotransmitters a psychoactive drug affects by examining its structure. Animal studies can add information about the specific areas of the brain in which the drug is active. Yet a full understanding of why a drug produces its individual effect and why closely related drugs have subtly different activities often remains tantalizingly out of reach.

Those gaps are especially evident concerning what is known about the psychedelic drugs. Most of these fascinating compounds have molecular structures with striking similarities to the amine neurotransmitters: dopamine, norepinephrine, and serotonin. There is evidence that they produce at least some of their effects by stimulating the activity of cells in the locus coeruleus — the brain center that integrates input about sensory perceptions — and the *raphe nucleus* — a part of the brain stem whose neurons connect with the emotion-controlling limbic system and other areas of the brain.

British author Aldous Huxley described mescaline's effect on him as a sensory overload that threatened his individual identity.

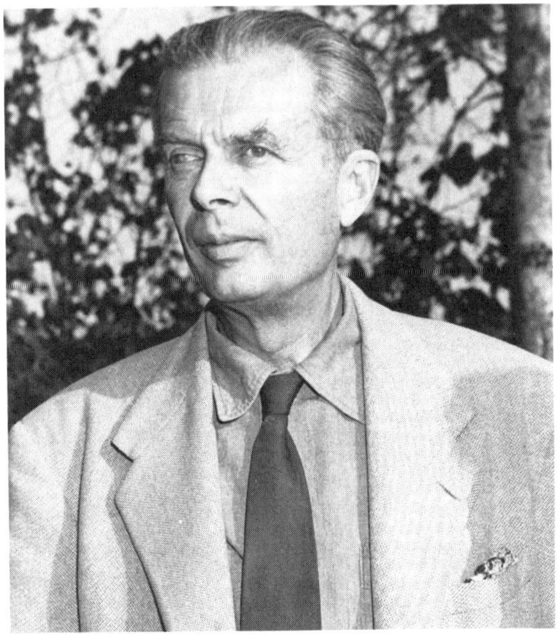

Synesthesia

Yet neuroscientists still cannot explain why psychedelic drugs have such vivid effects on a user's perception of the world. Users of some psychedelic drugs can experience a temporary feeling of unity with the universe — and can be plunged into terrifying psychoses. Scenes and sounds are distorted, sometimes pleasantly, sometimes not. The different senses may be intermingled in what is called *synesthesia*, so that a sound is "heard" as a color or "seen" as a visual effect. Time and space can expand unpredictably, so that minutes seem days long and a few feet seem to stretch for miles.

These experiences are not always enjoyable. When Aldous Huxley, the British author, took mescaline, he panicked at the feeling that his personality was "disintegrating under a pressure of reality greater than a mind accustomed to living most of the time in a cozy world of symbols could possibly bear." Users of other psychedelic drugs have attempted suicide because of the terror they felt or have been struck with schizophrenialike symptoms after a single drug-taking episode. And although many attempts have been made to use psychedelic drugs in medical treatment, the unpredictability and dangers of these substances have made such efforts unsuccessful.

Psychedelics and Ancient Religions

Although some of the drugs are very old, the word *psychedelic* is new. It was coined in the 1960s from the Greek word for "mind-manifesting" by a psychiatrist named Humphrey Osmond. The drugs are often called hallucinogens, but that name is not quite accurate. A hallucination is an imaginary experience, and the psychedelic drugs do not create such experiences. Instead, they distort customary perceptions.

Osmond said he chose the new name to include "the concepts of enriching the mind and enlarging the vision." Those concepts explain why some psychedelic drugs were incorporated in ancient religious practices. When the Spanish conquered Mexico, for example, they found that the Aztecs regarded the peyote cactus as sacred. A court physician who visited Mexico reported that "those who eat or chew it see visions either frightful or laughable." Peyote was a central part of the religion of the Mexican Indians, and its use was incorporated in their practice of Christianity. Peyotism was given official recognition in 1918 with the formation of the Native American Church of the United States, whose members use peyote legally in their rites.

Mescaline

The major active ingredient in the peyote cactus is mescaline. The chemical structure of mescaline was worked out in 1918. In the 1960s, Alexander Shulgin, a chemist with the Dow Chemical Company in California, began to synthesize modified versions of the mescaline molecule. In particular, he created a family of drugs called the *methoxyamphetamines*, which can be regarded as combinations of mescaline and amphetamines.

Earlier, we mentioned MDMA (Ecstasy) as an amphetamine analog. It can equally be regarded as a modification of mescaline, because it is a methoxyamphetamine. It has been used by some psychotherapists because of its apparent ability to enhance self-awareness. Another, more sinister methoxy-

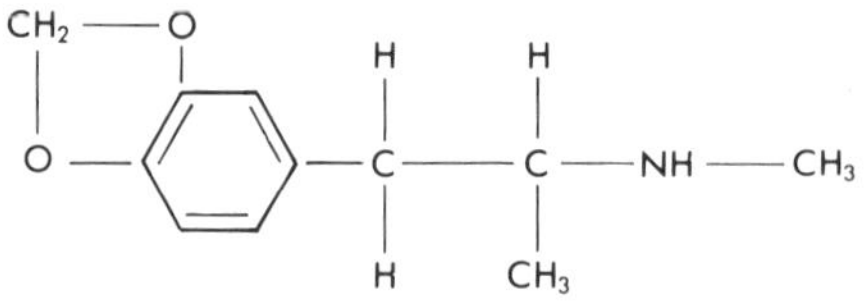

MDMA ("Ecstasy")

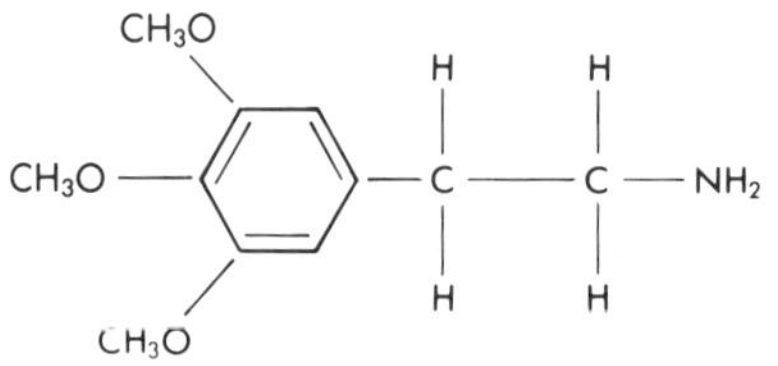

mescaline

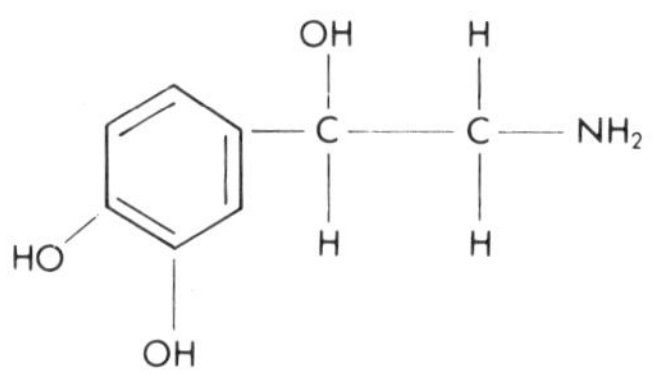

norepinephrine

Scientists believe that the reasons for the psychedelic effects of drugs such as LSD and mescaline may be attributable to the fact that they are molecularly similar to the neurotransmitters norepinephrine, serotonin, and dopamine.

amphetamine is DOM, known on the street as STP, which is more than 50 times as powerful as mescaline and is capable of causing frightening "bad trips." Like mescaline, the methoxyamphetamines have structures resembling that of norepinephrine, a point we shall return to later.

Psychedelic Mushrooms

Another psychoactive plant that was widely used in America when the Spanish arrived was the "magic mushroom," whose Indian name, *teonanacatl*, means "food of the gods." It too was commonly ingested to bring on visions during religious rites. It was not until the 1950s that samples of the magic mushroom were obtained by American scientists. It was identified as a member of the *Psilocybe* genus of mushrooms. In 1958 two active ingredients were isolated from the mushroom by Albert Hofmann, a chemist at the Sandoz Drug Company in Switzerland. Hofmann named them psilocybin and psilocin. The only difference between them is that psilocybin has a phosphorus atom that psilocin lacks. Structurally, both are similar to the neurotransmitter serotonin.

Lysergic Acid Diethylamide: LSD

Hofmann was asked to work on the magic mushroom because he was already famous for synthesizing the most notorious of psychedelic drugs, lysergic acid diethylamide, or LSD. The road to that synthesis started centuries ago, not with religious rites but with outbreaks of poisoning caused by rotten rye plants. A fungus called ergot can grow as a parasite on these plants. If the fungus is ingested, as happened often during medieval times, it can cause gangrene in the limbs serious enough to require amputation. But ergot has other effects that make it medically useful. It can accelerate childbirth by precipitating contraction of the uterus, and it also contracts blood vessels. Ergotamine, a chemical extracted from ergot, is the most effective treatment for migraine headaches, which are caused by expansion of blood vessels in the head. Another chemical that was isolated from ergot, ergonovine, causes the uterus to contract.

In the 1930s chemists at what was then the Rockefeller Institute of New York identified the chemical nucleus of the various compounds extracted from ergot. They named it lysergic acid. Hofmann used that discovery to develop a method for synthesizing large amounts of ergonovine for use in childbirth. Continuing his exploration of the ergot chemicals, Hofmann developed a mixture of three of them that is marketed under the trade name of Hydergine as a treatment for some mental conditions of the elderly, such as senility.

In Hofmann's methodical program, the 25th lysergic acid compound discovered was lysergic acid diethylamide, LSD-25. It was ignored for several years because it had no apparent effect on laboratory animals. But in 1943, acting on a hunch, Hofmann made a new batch of LSD-25. He had to stop work after accidentally ingesting some of the substance because, as he related the next day in a memorandum, of "a remarkable restlessness combined with a slight dizziness. At home I lay down and sank into a not unpleasant intoxicated-like condition characterized by an extremely stimulated imagination."

A few days later, Hofmann took what he thought was a small dose of the compound — a quarter of a milligram, which we now know to be close to an overdose. He described "demonic transformations of the outer world" so severe that at times he feared he was going insane or dying. It took him 14 hours to recover.

LSD was tried as a treatment for alcoholism and as an aid for terminal cancer patients to help them endure extreme pain, but a high incidence of "bad trips" ended those therapeutic efforts. LSD became notorious in the 1960s as a widely abused "recreational" drug. Its popularity faded as the drug's potential for severe psychotic reactions and even permanent damage to higher thought processes became evident.

Attempts to explain the psychedelic effects of all these drugs start with their molecular resemblance to the amine neurotransmitters serotonin, dopamine, and norepinephrine. LSD, psilocybin, and psilocin closely resemble serotonin, whereas mescaline has similarities to all three neurotransmitters. But research to pinpoint why the psychedelic drugs produce their unique effects has not made much progress.

LSD: Serotonin Antagonist

Much of what is known about the activity of psychedelic drugs has come from the work of George Aghajanian, a Yale University neuroscientist who has painstakingly measured the activity of serotonin neurons by inserting tiny electrodes into them.

Serotonin neurons in the brain were mapped in the 1960s by two Swedish researchers, Kjell Fuxe and Annica Dahlstrom, who found that they all originate from the group of brain stem structures called the raphe nuclei. Axons of neurons in the raphe nuclei extend to many parts of the brain, but a large number of them run to the limbic system.

In a series of experiments, Aghajanian injected mice with LSD and recorded the activity of serotonin neurons in their raphe nuclei. He found that an LSD injection inhibited the firing of the serotonin nuclei quickly and completely. Other neurons in the raphe nuclei were not affected. When Aghajanian ran the same experiments with other psychedelic drugs, he got mixed results. Some drugs, including psilocybin and psilocin, had the same effect as LSD. Others, including mescaline, did not. And lisuride, an LSD relative with no psychedelic powers, inhibited the serotonin neurons as effectively as LSD. So although one of LSD's properties is that it is a serotonin antagonist, this does not explain why it has the mind-altering effects that it does.

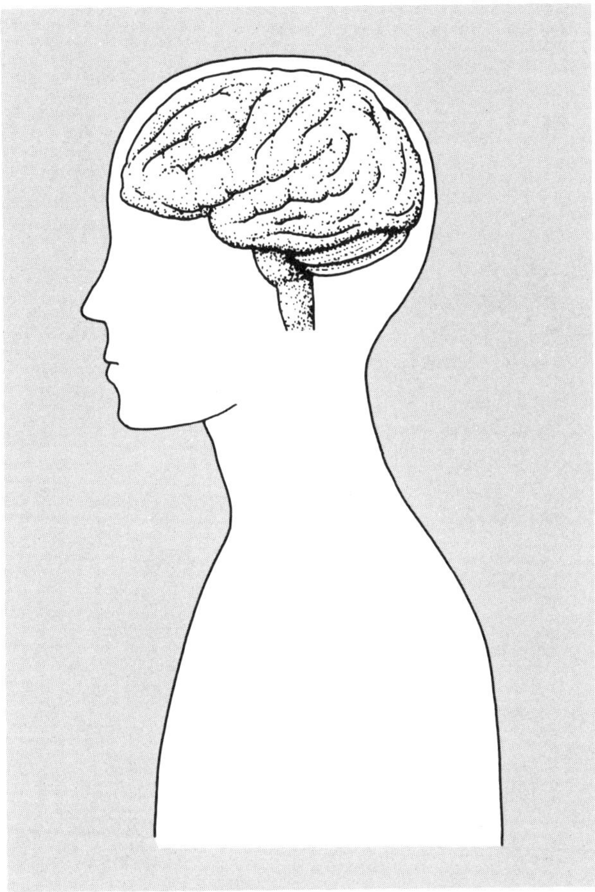

Ongoing studies concerning the ways drugs affect the human brain promise to lead to breakthroughs that will offer new perspectives on the mysteries of the human personality.

Psychedelics and Norepinephrine

Aghajanian has extended his experiments to norepinephrine neurons in the locus coeruleus. As was mentioned in Chapter 5, other researchers have shown that amphetamines increase the activity of these neurons by forcing norepinephrine out of the nerve endings. In animal experiments, Aghajanian first found that all sensory inputs, from sounds to odors to sights, make the neurons in the locus coeruleus fire faster. The rate of firing speeds up even more when the animal is given a psychedelic drug such as mescaline or LSD. Amphetamines do not accelerate the firing rate, nor do drugs that are structurally similar to LSD but produce no psychedelic activity.

Interestingly, psychedelic drugs do not speed up the firing rate of locus coeruleus neurons when there is no significant sensory input.

Aghajanian's work has moved us a step closer to an understanding of how psychedelic drugs work in the brain. Clearly, they stimulate the release of norepinephrine from neurons, much more than amphetamines do. The resulting spurt of brain-cell activity could account for the unusually heightened sense of self-awareness that psychedelic drugs often produce. The speedup of activity in the locus coeruleus, which integrates sensory messages from the eyes, ears, and other sense organs, could explain the phenomenon of synesthesia — sensing sound as colors, and so on. Presumably, the accelerated release of norepinephrine, and possibly other amine neurotransmitters, accounts for the psychotic reactions and bad trips that many psychedelic drug users report.

But there are still many unanswered questions. Aghajanian has shown that psychedelic drugs do not directly affect the locus coeruleus. Instead, they probably act on different neurons that in turn act on the locus coeruleus. Those neurons have not been identified yet, although some progress has been made in that direction. Several neuroscientists have found that psychedelic drugs act on a specific kind of serotonin receptor, called S2. A drug's effect on the S2 receptors is closely related to its psychedelic power in humans. A logical conclusion is that psychedelic drugs act on brain cells with S2 receptors, which act in turn on the locus coeruleus. The next step is to identify those S2-receptor neurons.

Keys to Human Nature

Since psychedelic drugs have no medical uses now, some might ask why this research is worth doing. One answer is that it opens a door through which we get a new view of the unique qualities of the human brain and the human personality. Over many decades, neuroscientists have worked out how the brain processes sensory information, identifying the specific pathways for signals from the eyes, ears, tongue, and other sensory organs. Research on psychedelic drugs is giving a broader view of how the brain handles the total sensory input. One message from this research seems to be that the locus coeruleus is at least partly responsible for our emotional response to what our eyes see and our ears hear.

Another message is that these drugs might enable us to come closer to an understanding of individual human personality. Psychedelic drugs seem to break down, at least temporarily, the barrier that separates the individual from the outside world, creating a sense of oneness with the universe. By learning how this happens, neuroscience will tell us more about how the brain creates a sense of individuality.

Step by step, research on psychoactive drugs is telling scientists more about the organization of the brain and the chemical basis of human behavior. They are learning how drugs such as the antidepressants and antianxiety agents can restore normality, how drugs such as the psychedelics can distort normal mental processes, and how drugs such as cocaine and the opiates can alter brain function. The dark side of this knowledge is the potential for the creation of drugs that can cause severe damage if they are misused. But in the right hands, knowledge about psychoactive drugs is leading to the discovery of new compounds that may be tomorrow's "miracle drugs" for the treatment of mental illness.

APPENDIX

State Agencies for the Prevention and Treatment of Drug Abuse

ALABAMA
Department of Mental Health
Division of Mental Illness and Substance Abuse Community Programs
200 Interstate Park Drive
P.O. Box 3710
Montgomery, AL 36193
(205) 271-9253

ALASKA
Department of Health and Social Services
Office of Alcoholism and Drug Abuse
Pouch H-05-F
Juneau, AK 99811
(907) 586-6201

ARIZONA
Department of Health Services
Division of Behavioral Health Services
Bureau of Community Services
Alcohol Abuse and Alcoholism Section
2500 East Van Buren
Phoenix, AZ 85008
(602) 255-1238

Department of Health Services
Division of Behavioral Health Services
Bureau of Community Services
Drug Abuse Section
2500 East Van Buren
Phoenix, AZ 85008
(602) 255-1240

ARKANSAS
Department of Human Services
Office on Alcohol and Drug Abuse Prevention
1515 West 7th Avenue
Suite 310
Little Rock, AR 72202
(501) 371-2603

CALIFORNIA
Department of Alcohol and Drug Abuse
111 Capitol Mall
Sacramento, CA 95814
(916) 445-1940

COLORADO
Department of Health
Alcohol and Drug Abuse Division
4210 East 11th Avenue
Denver, CO 80220
(303) 320-6137

CONNECTICUT
Alcohol and Drug Abuse Commission
999 Asylum Avenue
3rd Floor
Hartford, CT 06105
(203) 566-4145

DELAWARE
Division of Mental Health
Bureau of Alcoholism and Drug Abuse
1901 North Dupont Highway
Newcastle, DE 19720
(302) 421-6101

DISTRICT OF COLUMBIA

Department of Human Services
Office of Health Planning and
Development
601 Indiana Avenue, NW
Suite 500
Washington, D.C. 20004
(202) 724-5641

FLORIDA

Department of Health and
Rehabilitative Services
Alcoholic Rehabilitation Program
1317 Winewood Boulevard
Room 187A
Tallahassee, FL 32301
(904) 488-0396

Department of Health and
Rehabilitative Services
Drug Abuse Program
1317 Winewood Boulevard
Building 6, Room 155
Tallahassee, FL 32301
(904) 488-0900

GEORGIA

Department of Human Resources
Division of Mental Health and
Mental Retardation
Alcohol and Drug Section
618 Ponce De Leon Avenue, NE
Atlanta, GA 30365-2101
(404) 894-4785

HAWAII

Department of Health
Mental Health Division
Alcohol and Drug Abuse Branch
1250 Punch Bowl Street
P.O. Box 3378
Honolulu, HI 96801
(808) 548-4280

IDAHO

Department of Health and Welfare
Bureau of Preventive Medicine
Substance Abuse Section
450 West State
Boise, ID 83720
(208) 334-4368

ILLINOIS

Department of Mental Health and
Developmental Disabilities
Division of Alcoholism
160 North La Salle Street
Room 1500
Chicago, IL 60601
(312) 793-2907

Illinois Dangerous Drugs
Commission
300 North State Street
Suite 1500
Chicago, IL 60610
(312) 822-9860

INDIANA

Department of Mental Health
Division of Addiction Services
429 North Pennsylvania Street
Indianapolis, IN 46204
(317) 232-7816

IOWA

Department of Substance Abuse
505 5th Avenue
Insurance Exchange Building
Suite 202
Des Moines, IA 50319
(515) 281-3641

KANSAS

Department of Social Rehabilitation
Alcohol and Drug Abuse Services
2700 West 6th Street
Biddle Building
Topeka, KS 66606
(913) 296-3925

KENTUCKY
Cabinet for Human Resources
Department of Health Services
Substance Abuse Branch
275 East Main Street
Frankfort, KY 40601
(502) 564-2880

LOUISIANA
Department of Health and Human Resources
Office of Mental Health and Substance Abuse
655 North 5th Street
P.O. Box 4049
Baton Rouge, LA 70821
(504) 342-2565

MAINE
Department of Human Services
Office of Alcoholism and Drug Abuse Prevention
Bureau of Rehabilitation
32 Winthrop Street
Augusta, ME 04330
(207) 289-2781

MARYLAND
Alcoholism Control Administration
201 West Preston Street
Fourth Floor
Baltimore, MD 21201
(301) 383-2977

State Health Department
Drug Abuse Administration
201 West Preston Street
Baltimore, MD 21201
(301) 383-3312

MASSACHUSETTS
Department of Public Health
Division of Alcoholism
755 Boylston Street
Sixth Floor
Boston, MA 02116
(617) 727-1960

Department of Public Health
Division of Drug Rehabilitation
600 Washington Street
Boston, MA 02114
(617) 727-8617

MICHIGAN
Department of Public Health
Office of Substance Abuse Services
3500 North Logan Street
P.O. Box 30035
Lansing, MI 48909
(517) 373-8603

MINNESOTA
Department of Public Welfare
Chemical Dependency Program Division
Centennial Building
658 Cedar Street
4th Floor
Saint Paul, MN 55155
(612) 296-4614

MISSISSIPPI
Department of Mental Health
Division of Alcohol and Drug Abuse
1102 Robert E. Lee Building
Jackson, MS 39201
(601) 359-1297

MISSOURI
Department of Mental Health
Division of Alcoholism and Drug Abuse
2002 Missouri Boulevard
P.O. Box 687
Jefferson City, MO 65102
(314) 751-4942

MONTANA
Department of Institutions
Alcohol and Drug Abuse Division
1539 11th Avenue
Helena, MT 59620
(406) 449-2827

NEBRASKA

Department of Public Institutions
Division of Alcoholism and Drug Abuse
801 West Van Dorn Street
P.O. Box 94728
Lincoln, NB 68509
(402) 471-2851, Ext. 415

NEVADA

Department of Human Resources
Bureau of Alcohol and Drug Abuse
505 East King Street
Carson City, NV 89710
(702) 885-4790

NEW HAMPSHIRE

Department of Health and Welfare
Office of Alcohol and Drug Abuse Prevention
Hazen Drive
Health and Welfare Building
Concord, NH 03301
(603) 271-4627

NEW JERSEY

Department of Health
Division of Alcoholism
129 East Hanover Street CN 362
Trenton, NJ 08625
(609) 292-8949

Department of Health
Division of Narcotic and Drug Abuse Control
129 East Hanover Street CN 362
Trenton, NJ 08625
(609) 292-8949

NEW MEXICO

Health and Environment Department
Behavioral Services Division
Substance Abuse Bureau
725 Saint Michaels Drive
P.O. Box 968
Santa Fe, NM 87503
(505) 984-0020, Ext. 304

NEW YORK

Division of Alcoholism and Alcohol Abuse
194 Washington Avenue
Albany, NY 12210
(518) 474-5417

Division of Substance Abuse Services
Executive Park South
Box 8200
Albany, NY 12203
(518) 457-7629

NORTH CAROLINA

Department of Human Resources
Division of Mental Health, Mental Retardation and Substance Abuse Services
Alcohol and Drug Abuse Services
325 North Salisbury Street
Albemarle Building
Raleigh, NC 27611
(919) 733-4670

NORTH DAKOTA

Department of Human Services
Division of Alcoholism and Drug Abuse
State Capitol Building
Bismarck, ND 58505
(701) 224-2767

OHIO

Department of Health
Division of Alcoholism
246 North High Street
P.O. Box 118
Columbus, OH 43216
(614) 466-3543

Department of Mental Health
Bureau of Drug Abuse
65 South Front Street
Columbus, OH 43215
(614) 466-9023

OKLAHOMA
Department of Mental Health
Alcohol and Drug Programs
4545 North Lincoln Boulevard
Suite 100 East Terrace
P.O. Box 53277
Oklahoma City, OK 73152
(405) 521-0044

OREGON
Department of Human Resources
Mental Health Division
Office of Programs for Alcohol and Drug Problems
2575 Bittern Street, NE
Salem, OR 97310
(503) 378-2163

PENNSYLVANIA
Department of Health
Office of Drug and Alcohol Programs
Commonwealth and Forster Avenues
Health and Welfare Building
P.O. Box 90
Harrisburg, PA 17108
(717) 787-9857

RHODE ISLAND
Department of Mental Health, Mental Retardation and Hospitals
Division of Substance Abuse
Substance Abuse Administration Building
Cranston, RI 02920
(401) 464-2091

SOUTH CAROLINA
Commission on Alcohol and Drug Abuse
3700 Forest Drive
Columbia, SC 29204
(803) 758-2521

SOUTH DAKOTA
Department of Health
Division of Alcohol and Drug Abuse
523 East Capitol, Joe Foss Building
Pierre, SD 57501
(605) 773-4806

TENNESSEE
Department of Mental Health and Mental Retardation
Alcohol and Drug Abuse Services
505 Deaderick Street
James K. Polk Building, Fourth Floor
Nashville, TN 37219
(615) 741-1921

TEXAS
Commission on Alcoholism
809 Sam Houston State Office Building
Austin, TX 78701
(512) 475-2577

Department of Community Affairs
Drug Abuse Prevention Division
2015 South Interstate Highway 35
P.O. Box 13166
Austin, TX 78711
(512) 443-4100

UTAH
Department of Social Services
Division of Alcoholism and Drugs
150 West North Temple
Suite 350
P.O. Box 2500
Salt Lake City, UT 84110
(801) 533-6532

VERMONT
Agency of Human Services
Department of Social and Rehabilitation Services
Alcohol and Drug Abuse Division
103 South Main Street
Waterbury, VT 05676
(802) 241-2170

VIRGINIA
Department of Mental Health and Mental Retardation
Division of Substance Abuse
109 Governor Street
P.O. Box 1797
Richmond, VA 23214
(804) 786-5313

WASHINGTON
Department of Social and Health Service
Bureau of Alcohol and Substance Abuse
Office Building—44 W
Olympia, WA 98504
(206) 753-5866

WEST VIRGINIA
Department of Health
Office of Behavioral Health Services
Division on Alcoholism and Drug Abuse
1800 Washington Street East
Building 3 Room 451
Charleston, WV 25305
(304) 348-2276

WISCONSIN
Department of Health and Social Services
Division of Community Services
Bureau of Community Programs
Alcohol and Other Drug Abuse Program Office
1 West Wilson Street
P.O. Box 7851
Madison, WI 53707
(608) 266-2717

WYOMING
Alcohol and Drug Abuse Programs
Hathaway Building
Cheyenne, WY 82002
(307) 777-7115, Ext. 7118

GUAM
Mental Health & Substance Abuse Agency
P.O. Box 20999
Guam 96921

PUERTO RICO
Department of Addiction Control Services
Alcohol Abuse Programs
P.O. Box B-Y Rio Piedras Station
Rio Piedras, PR 00928
(809) 763-5014

Department of Addiction Control Services
Drug Abuse Programs
P.O. Box B-Y Rio Piedras Station
Rio Piedras, PR 00928
(809) 764-8140

VIRGIN ISLANDS
Division of Mental Health, Alcoholism & Drug Dependency Services
P.O. Box 7329
Saint Thomas, Virgin Islands 00801
(809) 774-7265

AMERICAN SAMOA
LBJ Tropical Medical Center
Department of Mental Health Clinic
Pago Pago, American Samoa 96799

TRUST TERRITORIES
Director of Health Services
Office of the High Commissioner
Saipan, Trust Territories 96950

Further Reading

Bolles, R.C. et al. "Endorphins and Behavior," in *Annual Review of Psychology*, vol. 33, 1983.

Christie, M.J. "Tolerance and Cross-Tolerance with Morphine Resulting from Physiological Release of Endogenous Opiates," in *Life Science*, vol. 31, no. 9, 1982.

Grinspoon, L., and Bakalar, J.B. *Cocaine*. New York: Basic Books, 1976.

Grinspoon, L., and Bakalar, J.B. *Psychedelic Drugs Reconsidered*. New York: Basic Books, 1979.

Lindesmith, A.R. *Addiction and Opiates*. Chicago: Aldine Publishing, 1968.

Snyder, S.H. *Drugs and the Brain*. New York: Scientific American Books, Inc., 1986.

Snyder, S.H. *Madness and the Brain*. New York: McGraw-Hill Book Company, 1974.

Glossary

addiction a condition caused by repeated drug use, characterized by a compulsive urge to continue using the drug, a tendency to increase the dosage, and physiological and/or psychological dependence

amygdala the part of the limbic system that, according to animal studies, is associated with control of anxiety

autonomic nervous system the part of the nervous system that is concerned with control of involuntary bodily functions

axons extensions of neurons; essential links that allow the neurons to communicate with one another

brain stem the lower part of the brain, which connects the forebrain and midbrain to the spinal cord

catecholamine a compound, such as dopamine or norepinephrine, that affects the nervous and cardiovascular systems, the metabolic rate, and body temperature

cerebral cortex the area of the brain that governs higher functions, such as thought and language

corpus striatum the area of the brain that regulates motor behavior

cross-tolerance tolerance to a drug that develops through continued use of another drug with similar pharmacological action

dendrite the branching extension of nerve cells; carries impulses toward the cell body

dopamine a neurotransmitter that acts, among other places, in the corpus striatum. Chemically, dopamine is a catecholamine

endorphins compounds produced in the brain that serve as the body's natural opiates; similar to enkephalins

ergot a fungus that grows on rye plants; can cause gangrene if ingested, but also has some medically useful effects

euphoria a mental high characterized by a sense of well-being

fetal alcohol syndrome a condition in which a mother's heavy drinking during pregnancy produces a specific set of physical and mental handicaps in her developing fetus. The symptoms include growth deficiency, a particular pattern of facial deformities, brain and spinal cord defects, and varying degrees of malfunctions in major organs

glia the non-nervous, or supporting, tissue of the brain and spinal cord

hormone a product of a living cell that is carried, as by the bloodstream, to other cells, which it stimulates by chemical action

inhibiting neurotransmitter a neurotransmitter that inhibits the firing of a neuron

limbic system a group of structures of the brain that are concerned with emotions and motivation

locus coeruleus literally, "dark-blue place"; a blue area of the brain stem that contains many norepinephrine receptors

medulla oblongata the part of the brain stem that controls breathing

neuron the fundamental functional unit of neural tissue

neurotoxin a poisonous compound that acts on the nervous system

neurotransmitter a chemical released by neurons that transmits nerve impulses across a synapse

norepinephrine a neurotransmitter found in the autonomic nervous system; chemically, norepinephrine is a catecholamine

opiates compounds from the milky juice of the poppy plant *Papaver somniferum*, including opium, morphine, codeine and their derivatives, such as heroin

opiate antagonist a drug that prevents an opiate from producing its characteristic effect

paranoid schizophrenia a mental disorder characterized by unwarranted feelings of persecution

physical dependence adaption of the body to the presence of a drug such that its absence produces withdrawal symptoms

psychological dependence a condition in which the drug user craves a drug to maintain a sense of well-being and feels discomfort when deprived of it

receptor a specialized component of a cell that combines with a chemical substance to alter the function of the cell; for example, nerve-cell receptors combine with neurotransmitters

substantia gelatinosa center in the brain where pain nerves make their first contact with the spinal cord

sulci valleys on the surface of the cerebral cortex; they become wider in cases of brain atrophy

sympathetic nervous system a division of the autonomic nervous system that regulates such activities as hormone secretion and heartbeat

synapse the narrow gap between neurons; the point at which a nerve impulse is transmitted from one neuron to another

thalamus the part of the brain that receives pain messages and then relays them to other parts of the brain

tolerance a decrease of susceptibility to the effects of a drug due to its continued administration, resulting in the user's need to increase the drug dosage in order to achieve the effects experienced previously

withdrawal the physiological and psychological effects of discontinued use of a drug

Picture Credits

AP/Wide World Photos: pp. 75, 79; Art Resource: p. 81; Marion Bernstein/Art Resource: p. 58; The Bettmann Archive: pp. 10, 20, 32, 36, 37, 45; Bilarchiv Foto Marburg/Art Resource: p. 50; DEA: p. 74; EPA/Art Resource: p. 84; James Hamilton, Village Voice: p. 72; The Johns Hopkins Medical Institutions: p. 12; The Fitzhugh Ludlow Memorial Library: pp. 60, 67; New York Academy of Medicine Library: pp. 18, 48; New York Public Library Picture Collection: p. 27; Courtesy of R.E. Schultes: p. 62; United Nations: pp. 30, 35; UN Photo: p. 40; UPI/Bettmann Newsphotos: pp. 42, 53, 65, 70, 77, 86; The Upjohn Co.: p. 8.

Gary Tong Original Illustrations: pp. 21, 24, 28, 38, 57, 66, 68, 88, 91.

Index

Edward Edelson is the Science Editor of the New York Daily News and the past president of the National Association of Science Writers. He is the author of a number of books, including the forthcoming *Woman's Guide to Prescription Narcotics.* He has published extensively in magazines and journals on topics in medicine and science.

Solomon H. Snyder, M.D. is Distinguished Service Professor of Neuroscience, Pharmacology and Psychiatry at The Johns Hopkins University School of Medicine. He has served as president of the Society for Neuroscience and in 1978 received the Albert Lasker Award in Medical Research. He has authored *Uses of Marijuana, Madness and the Brain, The Troubled Mind, Biological Aspects of Mental Disorder,* and edited *Perspective in Neuropharmacology: A Tribute to Julius Axelrod.* Professor Snyder was a research associate with Dr. Axelrod at the National Institutes of Health.

Barry L. Jacobs, Ph.D., is currently a professor in the program of neuroscience at Princeton University. Professor Jacobs is author of *Serotonin Neurotransmission and Behavior* and *Hallucinogens: Neurochemical, Behavioral and Clinical Perspectives.* He has written many journal articles in the field of neuroscience and contributed numerous chapters to books on behavior and brain science. He has been a member of several panels of the National Institute of Mental Health.

Joann Ellison Rodgers, M.S. (Columbia), became Deputy Director of Public Affairs and Director of Media Relations for the Johns Hopkins Medical Institutions in Baltimore, Maryland, in 1984 after 18 years as an award-winning science journalist and widely read columnist for the Hearst newspapers.